Music, Culture, and the Politics of Health

Music, Culture, and the Politics of Health

Ethnography of a South African AIDS Choir

Austin C. Okigbo

LEXINGTON BOOKS
Lanham • Boulder • New York • London

Published by Lexington Books
An imprint of The Rowman & Littlefield Publishing Group, Inc.
4501 Forbes Boulevard, Suite 200, Lanham, Maryland 20706
www.rowman.com

Unit A, Whitacre Mews, 26-34 Stannary Street, London SE11 4AB

British Library Cataloguing in Publication Information Available

Library of Congress Cataloging-in-Publication Data
Names: Okigbo, Austin C., author.
Title: Music, culture, and the politics of health : ethnography of a South African AIDS choir / Austin C. Okigbo.
Description: Lanham, Maryland : Lexington Books [2016] | Includes bibliographical references and index.
Identifiers: LCCN 2016024304 (print) | LCCN 2016024670 (ebook) | ISBN 9781498510103 (cloth : alk. paper) | ISBN 9781498510110 (Electronic)
Subjects: LCSH: Music—Social aspects—South Africa. | AIDS (Disease)—South Africa. | Siphithemba Choir.
Classification: LCC ML3917.S62 O4 2016 (print) | LCC ML3917.S62 (ebook) | DDC 306.4/8420968—dc23
LC record available at https://lccn.loc.gov/2016024304

∞™ The paper used in this publication meets the minimum requirements of American National Standard for Information Sciences—Permanence of Paper for Printed Library Materials, ANSI/NISO Z39.48-1992.

Printed in the United States of America

Msgr. Theophilus Okere*, my initial inspirator in choral music; and late* ***Fr. Peter Njoku****, who remained my friend and mentor until his passing in 2006; just about the time I was getting ready for the initial phase of the research that culminated in this book.*

Contents

List of Illustrations

List of Tables

List of Abbreviations

ABC	*Abstain, Be faithful, Condomize*
AIDS	*acquired immuno deficiency syndrome*
AME	*African Methodist Episcopal* [*Church*]
anc	*antenatal clinic*
ANC	*African National Congress*
ARHAP	*African Religious Health Assets Programme*
ART	*antiretroviral therapy*
ARV	*antiretroviral*
ASSECA	*Association for the Educational and Cultural Development of the African People*
BCM	*Black Consciousness Movement*
CAPRISA	*Center for the AIDS Programme of Research in South Africa*
CBD	*commercial and business district*
CD4	*cluster designation 4 (a protein molecule in human blood)*
COSATU	*Congress of the South African Trade Unions*
DA	*Democratic Alliance*
HBCU	*historical Black colleges and universities*
HIV	*human immunodeficiency virus*
ICU	*Industrial and Commercial Workers' Union*
IDAMASA	*Interdenominational Association of African Ministers of Religion*
ILAM	*International Library of African Music*
KZN	*KwaZulu-Natal*
MRC	*Medical Research Council* [*of South Africa*]
NEPAD	*New Partnership for African Development*
OVC	*orphans and vulnerable children*
PAC	*Pan-African Congress*
PACSA	*Pietermaritzburg Agency for Christian Social Awareness*

PARC	*Partnership for AIDS Research Center*
PEPFAR	*President's Emergency Plan for AIDS Relief*
PLWA	*people living with [HIV and] AIDS*
SABC	*South African Broadcasting Corporation*
SAFM	*South African frequency modulation [radio]*
SANAC	*South African National AIDS Council*
SASO	*South African Student Organization*
STD	*sexually transmitted disease*
STI	*sexually transmitted infection*
TAC	*treatment action campaign*
TB	*tuberculosis*
UKZN	*University of KwaZulu-Natal*
UN	*United Nations*
UNAIDS	*United Nations Programme on HIV/AIDS*
UNICEF	*United Nations International Children's Emergency Fund*
USAID	*United States Agency for International Development*
WCC	*World Council of Churches*
WHO	*World Health Organization*

Note on Zulu Orthography and Diction

The orthographic model presented here is drawn from Compact Zulu Dictionary: English–Zulu, Zulu–English, compiled by G. R. Dent and edited by C. L. S. Nyembezi (Pietermaritzburg: Shuter & Shooter, [1959] 2002).

a = as in the English word *bark* (e.g., *Shaka,* the Zulu founding monarch)
e = as in the English word *bed* (e.g., *ihele* 'row of people')
i = as in the English word *feast,* (e.g., *biza* 'to call')
o = two sounds: an "open" sound, as in English *ball* (e.g., *ibhola* 'ball') and a "closed" sound, as in English *coat* (e.g., *isigodi* 'ravine')
u = as in the English word *fool* (e.g., *imbuzi* 'goat')

SELECT CONSONANTS

bh = "hard" *b,* as in the English word *bed* (e.g., *ibhanoyi* 'airplane')
c = a click sound, resembling an expression of exasperation, made by pressing the tip of the tongue against the forepart of the upper mouth, and suddenly withdrawing it (e.g., *cela* 'to ask')
ch = an aspirated sound of *c* (e.g., *ichibi* 'pond')
dl = combined voiced consonants (e.g., *dlala* 'to play')
gc = combined voiced sounds of English *g* and Zulu *ce* (e.g., *gcaba* 'to vaccinate')
gx = combined voiced sounds of English *g* and Zulu *x* (e.g., *imigxala* 'crow bars')
kh = an aspirated sound, as in English word *car* (e.g., *khala* 'to cry')
kl = combined voiced consonants of English *k* and *l* (e.g., *klwebah* 'to scratch')

ng = as in the English word *linger,* but never as in *ginger* (e.g., *Ohlange,* the location of John L. Dube's Zulu Ohlange Institute)
ph = an aspirated English *p,* but never as in *phone* (e.g., *phata* 'to hold')
q = a click sound, produced by pressing the front part of the tongue against the pallet, and then releasing the tongue sharply (e.g., *qamba* 'to make up')
qh = the aspirated sound of the click *q* (e.g., *qhamuka* 'to appear')
sh = as in the English word *should* (e.g., *shayeli* 'driver')
th = the aspirated sound of English *t,* but never as in *thing* (e.g., *thatha* 'to take')
tsh= a more ejective sound of the start of the English word *cheek* (e.g., *utshwala* 'beer')
x = a click sound, similar to the sound made to urge a horse to greater speed (e.g,. *ixoxo* 'frog')
xh = the aspirated sound of the click sound of *x* (e.g., *xhuma* 'to join together')

Acknowledgments

I began the research that led to this book project a few years ago as a Fulbright fellow in South Africa. Upon completing my doctoral dissertation I continued to work on the topic, following up on issues related to HIV and AIDS in South Africa, Africa, and on the global scene. I maintained contact with the Siphithemba Choir, and later made a number of subsequent trips between 2011 through 2013, including a concert tour with the Williams College Chamber Choir in the winter of 2012 during which, under the joint leadership with my colleague Brad Wells, we had inspiring collaborative concerts with the Siphithemba Choir in Durban. I met and interacted with different individuals and organizations during these years that helped me to understand the language of health in general and HIV/AIDS in particular, knowledge that allowed me to appreciate the problem at a much deeper level so as to effectively contextualize the music of AIDS within the subtleties of the history, culture, and politics of health at local and global levels. Therefore the research and the process that gave birth to this book project is owing to a number of persons as well as enabling environment in different places and institutions that afforded me the time and space to gather and to sort through the data, and the resources to do the actual writing of this book.

First I thank the Lord, who graciously lavished me with the strength of body and mind to accomplish this study. I also thank my local ordinary, Archbishop A. J. V. Obinna of the Catholic Archdiocese of Owerri, Nigeria for the initial opportunity of institutional music training. To the Siphithemba Choir, I offer thanks for working with me. This work is about them, but it is also for them and on their behalf.

Various institutions contributed in different ways to facilitate this undertaking and ultimately make this book project possible: the United States Department of Education; the United States Consulate in Durban, and the United

States Embassy at Pretoria, which supported my stay in South Africa; the Alan Paton Center and Struggle Archives at the Pietermaritzburg Campus of the University of KwaZulu-Natal (UKZN); the UKZN Theology Department, Pietermaritzburg Campus; the Opera Studio and Choral Academy at UKZN in Durban; the Diakonia Council of Churches; the Pietermaritzburg Agency for Christian Social Awareness; the Nkosinathi Project at the Emmanuel Cathedral, and the Archdiocese of Durban; KwaMashu Community Resource Center; St. Clement Home-Based Care Project; and the Clermont Community Resource Center.

I am indebted to individual friends in South Africa who helped in different ways to make my research a success, especially Mrs. S. Mlambo who gave me easy access to much valuable information at the Home-based Care Project that she managed at the St. Clement Catholic Church in Clermont as well as introduced me to many individuals who pointed me in the right direction for information. Thanks to her work and with the immense support of her daughter and my friend Dr. Phumzile Mlambo-Ngcuka, former Deputy President of South Africa and currently the Under-Secretary-General of the United Nations and the Executive Director of UN Women, the lives of many women, AIDS orphans and vulnerable children were saved and improved for better. Dr. Mlambo-Ngcuka's current appointment at the United Nations is a testimony to her commitment to the welfare of women and children. I am equally indebted to my friend Muziwandile Hadebe and family, Father Steve Tully, the administrator of Emmanuel Cathedral, Fr. Peter Sodje C.S.Sp, and Constance Sediyadiya.

What would eventually set the stage for this book began at Indiana University, Bloomington thanks to my mentors who continued to encourage me to pursue this book project: Professors Ruth M. Stone, Mellonee Burnim, Portia Maultsby, Daniel Reed, and Judah Cohen. I am equally thankful to a host of family friends from Bloomington whose love and support cannot be overstated. Professor Osita Afoaku and Dr. Oyibo Afoaku and their family are invaluable in their love and support. A number of friends who were fellow students have maintained very strong and supportive relationships with me including Boubacar Diakite who is now at Harvard and his family, Juliet Glenn-Callender, Gillian Richards-Greaves and her family, Sr. Immaculate Kyampeire, Ebrima Diallo and family; Eduardo Wolf and his wife Jill and family; Majid and Fatima Al-Harthy and family; Amina McIntyre, and Jolanta Mickute, Paul Schauert and Jennifer Hart, Violet Naanyu, and a host of other African and African American students.

My life here at the University of Colorado, Boulder has been a very pleasant one since I joined the faculty a few years ago thanks to strong support and mentorship from my colleagues in the college of music and ethnic studies. HIV/AIDS research is so fleeting that it requires regular updating of data. For this I am grateful to the office of the provost and dean emeritus Dan Sher who provided me the kind of initial financial support that allowed me to return to South Africa a few times to update my data, thus enabling me to present my recent findings at conferences and to complete the book manuscript.

Finally, I thank my family for the support I have received from them all these years. I commend to God in prayer my father, who passed into God's glory at the beginning of this research. I am especially thankful for my mother Florence Okigbo, and my siblings Lucy Unakalamba and family, Chris, Nathaniel, Emma, Vita Okigbo and their families, Jane Akobueze and Augustina Okere and their families for their health, love, and faith.

I cannot finish without offering thanks for Fr. Michael Okere, my brother and friend here in the U.S. Fr. Levi Nkwocha, and Mrs. Immaculata Amanze and family. Sr. Bellarmine Ezumah, who is a professor at Murray State University, Kentucky has been a wonderful and intellectually inspiring friend. Professor Paul Nnodim of the Massachusetts College of the Liberal Arts has been a wonderful brother and colleague. Thank you for all your support and patience with reading through my work whenever I call on you.

Other people who I must mention for their love and care since the time I got here in Colorado are Fr. Gabriel Okafor, the families of Dr. and Mrs. Ikwuakor, Mr. and Mrs. Cosmas Agwu, Mr. and Mrs. C. Idika, Mr. and Mrs. Tunde Johnson and the entire Johnson family, and Chief and Mrs. John O. Idowu. To the Nigerian and African Catholic communities at St. Ignatius Loyola, Denver and Queen of Peace, Aurora, I remain indebted for their continued love and spiritual support. Several loved ones and friends have touched my life and have silently contributed to making this undertaking worthwhile. I am indebted to them, and I offer thanks for their love and support.

Chapter 1

Introduction

Toward Ethnography of AIDS Music in a South African Experience

I finished attending mass at the Emmanuel Cathedral on a sunny Sunday afternoon and called up my friend Muzi to give me a ride to Umlazi, a Black township in the Greater Durban area of KwaZulu-Natal, also deemed the second largest after Soweto in the Guateng Province. My Toyota Conquest had developed a gearbox problem during the week, and it would remain at the auto shop at the Overport for a few days. Meanwhile, I had scheduled to meet with the Siphithemba Choir on this day for the first time. In Durban during the week, I had met Phumlani Kunene, its conductor, and Xolani Zulu, a choir member and the founder of the African Vision Shop on West Street. Phumlani had told me he would inform the choir members about my visit, and had asked that I endeavor to be at their rehearsal at 4:30 p.m. that Sunday.

Muzi, his son Lwandile. I arrived at Umlazi at about 5:00 p.m. A young man led us into Sizwe's yard through an old, narrow wooden gate on a rusty, shoulder level, wire gauze fence. I could immediately hear the choir singing. Their sound was coming from the garage right in front of the house. One of the garage doors was closed, while the other was lifted midway. Sizwe was rehearsing the choir, and Xolani was singing in the choir, but Phumlani was not there. Xolani offered us a seat on a long bench in front of the choir and quickly returned to singing with the group. For the next hour, the choir performed several songs, many of which were performed over a sound track from an amplified CD player. I listened carefully, and watched with keen interest the intensity of their dance moves and the air of camaraderie that surrounded their style of performance. It was a cold winter afternoon, and Muzi and I were dressed very warmly, but the choir members were sweating profusely from the heavy lifting of feet of the Zulu traditional dance.

I did not understand everything the choir sang on the first day that I heard it, but I noted the themes that were expressed in the music. These included love, fidelity, the Black race, and Africa. Love and fidelity in the context of HIV/AIDS made immediate sense to me, but terms like *abantu abamnyama* and *abansundu* "Black people" and "Black race" and *Africa* became clear only as my work with the group progressed. I came to appreciate the choir's take on the private and public discourse of HIV/AIDS. Apparently, the choir has positioned itself to engage in a struggle that is ideologically similar to that witnessed under apartheid. Issues of race, Africa in the global politics of AIDS, the politics of culture and identity, economic and social justice, and the role of faith, comprise the tapestry of ideas that define Siphithemba's worldview, and these are articulated and expressed in the choir's organizing and performing. They also comprise the issues that I dealt with throughout the course of this study, issues that I address extensively in this work.

THE HIV/AIDS AS PUBLIC HEALTH ISSUE IN SOUTH AFRICA

The year 1990 marked a new beginning in the history of modern South Africa. In that year, F. W. de Klerk, the new president, lifted the ban on political organizations, including the African National Congress (ANC) and the Pan-African Congress (PAC), and announced the release of Nelson Mandela from prison. Parliament repealed the Separate Amenities Act and lifted the nationwide state of emergency, a legal fiction that had enabled the suppression of resistance movements. These changes marked the beginning of an end to more than five hundred years of political, economic, cultural, and social subjugation of Africans in the land by Europeans—a period that had begun with the arrival of the first Portuguese merchants on the southernmost tip of the continent in 1488 (Worden 1994). The subjugation had reached its apogee with the institutionalization of the apartheid ('aparthood, apartness') system by the Afrikaner-led Nationalist Party in 1948. The oppression inflicted by this system saw Africans engage in decades of struggle for freedom and human rights, culminating in the transition to majority democratic rule, in which Nelson Mandela became the first Black president of South Africa.

Shortly after the total repealing of the apartheid laws with the inauguration of the new constitution in 1996, and the beginning of a period that ushered in a new light of hope and the restoration of the dignity of a people who had seen centuries of oppression, South Africans would face a dire public health situation in the HIV/AIDS pandemic, which forced a new conversation on the meanings of freedom, social and economic justice, human dignity, and human rights in general. As South Africa nears a quarter of century of popular democracy, HIV/AIDS continues to comprise a major public health concern.

Although the UNAIDS *Global Report* shows "historic declines in AIDS-related deaths and new HIV infections and the mobilization of unprecedented financing for HIV-related activities in low- and middle-income countries" (2013: 2), the latest South African National HIV Prevalence, Incidence, and Behavior Survey released on April 1, 2014 shows that over 12.2% (i.e., over six million) of the population is HIV-positive. The survey, which is conducted by the Human Sciences Research Council in collaboration with a number of other international agencies including UNICEF and the Bill and Melinda Gates Foundation, indicates a 2% rise from the last survey that was conducted in 2008. The highest prevalence according to the UNAIDS report is in the age bracket 15-49 at 18%. The UN reports also indicates over 240, 000 deaths in 2012 alone, resulting in over 2.5 million orphans and vulnerable children between ages 0 and 17. The African population still maintains the highest prevalence over all. According to the HSRC report released in 2014, the prevalence in the African population is highest among Black African females aged 20–34 years. The next most-at-risk groups being Black African males aged 25–49 years. Each of these groups according to the HSRC report has HIV prevalence rate above 30% (2014: 53).

The general provincial prevalence based on the same HSRC study puts KwaZulu-Natal (KZN) where I have been conducting research since 2007 on top of the national statistical chart, translating the figure to more than two million people living with HIV and AIDS. Hence the province is still considered the center of the national HIV/AIDS prevalence.

I conducted this research in the Greater Durban area, including the townships of KwaMashu, Clermont, KwaMakutha, and Umlazi. I visited and observed activities in community-resource centers and home-based care projects, including the St. Clement Catholic Parish Clermont, KwaMashu Community Resource Center at the G2 Methodist Church, and the Nkosinathi Project at the Emmanuel Roman Catholic Cathedral in Durban. Since the resource centers kept statistical data on how many people they had cared for, I was curious to see if there were observable indications of an upward or downward turn in the HIV/AIDS cases. My aim was to see to what extent the data on the local communities where I worked were consistent with the province-wide statistics. These data provided a perspective on the nature of the problem in the area and enabled me to appreciate the effect of community-based projects in combating the epidemic. The latest data that I examined at the various centers during my last visit between 2012 and 2013 are very consistent with HSRC report on the following levels: that the rate of new infections and deaths has dropped generally thanks to wider distribution of the ARV, which means that people are living longer. However the highest number of new cases is reported among young adults between the ages of 20 and 30 years, which account for the majority of new infections in the population. The rise in new infections among the age bracket is explained by the report as being a result of the plunge in the use of condoms, less than 68%

compared to 85% between 2008 and 2010; exponential rise (23%) among people with multiple sex partners especially among adult males; decline in HIV public awareness; and environmental factors such as continued rise in informal (squatter) settlements around the urban centers with limited to no adequate sanitary conditions.

Another aspect of the statistics that showed consistency in the centers since I began my documentation is the steady number of patients who reported other ailments particularly tuberculosis. In most cases, tuberculosis patients were categorized as TB+, an indication that they were HIV/AIDS-positive persons with tuberculosis. They represent a dire local public health situation with regard to complications arising from opportunistic infections, especially tuberculosis. In fact, in 2007, the provincial minister for health in KwaZulu-Natal announced over the radio that the rate of tuberculosis (and its extreme drug-resistant strain, XDR) in the province was already at level of a pandemic. What was particularly troubling about the situation was the rate of the prevalence of HIV/AIDS and tuberculosis among Africans in the communities in which I worked, the province, and in the country as a whole. Based on personal observation, the current situation of XDR is not showing signs of abating.

Having concluded in their report that there is substantial increase in HIV prevalence in South Africa (2014: 124–128), the HSRC recommended "evidence-based, diversified, and comprehensive multi-sectoral response to the HIV and AIDS epidemic" (129–131). One question then this work seeks to answer is how a choral group of HIV-positive individuals through their musical activities comprise part of the "multi-sectoral" approach in their response to the HIV/AIDS and health situation in their community.

SOUTH AFRICA'S CREATIVE AND EXPRESSIVE RESPONSES TO THE HIV/AIDS SITUATION

The pre-1994 government response to HIV/AIDS has been largely described as ineffectual (Seftel 1988: 17–22). First, the political upheaval of the 1980s and the preoccupation with the transformations and transition to democracy in the early 1990s distracted the government from formulating a policy that would effectively have addressed the HIV/AIDS crisis. Second, the belief that HIV was an exclusively White homosexual problem influenced the Department of National Health and Population Development to establish AIDS-training, information, and counseling centers only in the major White urban areas, starting in 1988 (Nattrass 2007: 38). A major public-policy development on AIDS came in 1996, when President Nelson Mandela declared the HIV/AIDS pandemic "the next struggle" (Ndungane 2003: 58). Further robust public policies, though marred by controversies, were implemented under the administration of President Thabo Mbeki, who, with his health minister, Manto Tshabalala-Nsimang, was widely criticized for denying that HIV causes AIDS. In the opinion of many critics, the incoherence and ineffectuality of the government's AIDS policy was seemingly built on such denialism.[1]

Nelson Mandela's declaration of HIV/AIDS as "the next struggle" was symbolic, but also significant because of the temporal proximity between apartheid and the explosion of the AIDS epidemic, and the general understanding that the lingering effects of apartheid, namely the "unjust conditions of poverty and underdevelopment contributed substantially to the spread of HIV" (Vitillo 1991: 3). Similarly, in the *Oikos Journey* document issued in 2006 by the Diakonia Council of Churches in Durban, the ecumenical body declared, "in a context of a pandemic of HIV/AIDS and massive inequality, we can and must talk about poverty—and so we can and must engage with economics" (2006: 23).

The discursive linking of HIV/AIDS with the story of apartheid is consistent with the daily discourses on problems of the present dispensations in South Africa, which constantly reference history. This referencing is perhaps best summed up in the words of the renowned South African playwright and social critic Zakes Mda, who wrote in a preface to John Kani's *Nothing but the Truth,* "the past will always be a powerful presence in the present. . . . For those of us who are survivors of the past, it is important that we do not forget" (2002). The key element here is the power of the past. This understanding permeates public discourse on HIV/AIDS. Hence the sentiment generated by Mandela's linking of the two issues now permeates many of the facets of the AIDS discourse in South Africa, and a segment of the civil society that has succeeded in making this link in powerful ways is that of artists, cartoonists, and musicians who have employed symbolic imageries in their expressive and performance forms to inform, educate, and to communicate to their audiences messages that hinge on the war against HIV/AIDS (Bourgault 2003: xxv). A few examples illustrate this stance. First is the picture of a blood-soaked dying twelve-year-old Hector Peterson carried by Mbuyisa Makhubo accompanied by Hector's wailing sister, Antoinette, which became a dominant image of the antiapartheid struggles. Sam Nzima took the picture on 16 June 1976 during the Soweto student uprising. Hector had been gunned down by the apartheid police force. In a poster for the campaign for access to antiretroviral drugs, the South African Treatment Action Campaign juxtaposed this image with the image of another twelve-year-old, Nkosi Johnson, the AIDS victim and activist who spoke at the thirteenth international AIDS conference in Durban. At the conference, Nkosi pleaded with his government to make antiretroviral treatments available to HIV/AIDS patients. He died a few months later, leaving a legacy of activism through outspokenness, which continues to be invoked. In the poster, Hector Peterson's image is titled "June 16, 1976. Hector Peterson. Age 12"; the juxtaposed image is titled "June 1, 2001. Nkosi Johnson. Age 12." The poster thus draws a parallel between the two historical realities, unequivocally indicting the regime of then president Thabo Mbeki in its inaction for the death of the modern twelve-year-old, a victim of a long history that had claimed the life of another twelve-year-old, some twenty-five years before. In 2006, Valo, the political cartoonist for the *Soweto Times,* adapted Hector Peterson's image in a cartoon titled "Nkosi Johnson 1989–2001. Champion of the New Struggle." Similarly, the *Mail & Guardian* cartoonist Jonathan Shapiro, popularly known as Zapiro from his cartoon signature, adapted the same image of Hector Peterson and labeled it "The New Struggle" while inscribing "HIV/AIDS" on what was supposed to be Hector's blood-drenched school jersey. Valo and Zapiro conflated two historical experiences—apartheid and HIV/AIDS—and effectively made them one issue. This sense of the present experience of the HIV/AIDS pandemic has become a major component of the public discourse on HIV/AIDS in South Africa.

Another symbolic linking of HIV/AIDS with apartheid is the annual world music concert of musicians that is organized by the Nelson Mandela Foundation for HIV/AIDS treatment and prevention. The concert, nicknamed 46664, Mandela's prison number on Roben Island, aims to raise awareness and funds to provide treatment and care for HIV-positive persons in Africa and orphans and vulnerable children. This is in line with Mandela's declaration in that HIV/AIDS now constitutes the "new struggle" (Ndungane 2003: 58). The declaration that HIV/AIDS now constitutes a "new struggle" started a new conversation, which looked at the experience of the human struggles in South Africa, especially under apartheid, as having present effects with regard to HIV and AIDS. Naming the concert after Mandela's prison number symbolizes the new struggle, which carries in it a vision and hope of future successful defeat of the disease, just like the hope that saw Mandela through his years of incarceration, into his triumph in the final achievement of freedom for all peoples in South Africa.

At the beginning of this research, I became aware through a SABC television program that the number 46664 had been adopted by activists who sought to use the 20-20 Cricket World Cup (one of different types of cricket tournaments) that was held in South Africa in 2007 to raise awareness and advocate for HIV/AIDS treatment. Similar techniques have also been documented at cricket games in 2009 and 2010 respectively. In cricket, hitting 4 and 6 points, out of the field of play and out of the park respectively, are results of excellent batting, which could put a team ahead of its opponents. Thus, in the game of cricket, 4 and 6 are considered favorable numbers. At the games, fans carry and raise numbers 4 and 6 when they want to encourage the batting team to hit long shots. AIDS activists therefore choreographed the use of the numbers by placing members in the crowd who occasionally raised 4-6-6-6-4 to the cameras, with the intention of drawing people's attention to what the number newly symbolized. Just as the number once symbolized struggle against and victory over apartheid, so now it denoted the "new struggle," as had been declared by the man who had borne that number in prison during the previous struggle. The numbers may represent a long shot in the game of cricket, but so was the seeming long shot during the struggles that defeated apartheid and gained freedom and equality for all.

On the musical front, I documented between several instances in which songs drawn from the antiapartheid struggles were adapted to fit with the current experience of the HIV/AIDS. During one of my visits in South Africa for example, I documented a chorus performed by the participants at the South African AIDS Foundation Retreat in Durban

There is a race that I must run
Yes, a victory to be won
Give me power, any hour
Through and through

This song belongs in the category of songs called *amakhorasi,* which are normally short texts rendered to simple repetitive melodies, normally in rudimentary call-and-response pattern. Michael Ngqolowa, then Regional Secretary General of the Congress of South African Trade Unions (COSATU) and member of the ANC youth league however confirmed that the song would belong among those that could more naturally and spontaneously be appropriated in street demonstrations during the 1980s and 1990s. Now adapted in the context of the HIV/AIDS experience, the song's eschatological vision -the theological concept of End Times, the Last Judgment and Heaven and Hell- was transformed to convey visions of hope in the fight against HIV/AIDS.

Another song example was performed by Rev. Mandla Mdabe a Methodist minister, during an AIDS awareness event at St. Clement Catholic Church in Claremont near Durban. Rev. Mdabe who lives positively, and is well know for his motivational speeches around KwaZulu-Natal intoned a recognizable *toyi toyi* song that was commonly used in street demonstrations in the townships during the 1980s and early 1990s thus:

This fight needs a gun,
Give me a gun and I will shoot the Boer.

Rev. Mdabe altered the text of the song to suite the purpose of AIDS thus:

This fight needs a condom,
If we use the condom, we will defeat AIDS.

In October 2007, during a candlelight service that was organized by the Diakonia Council of Churches in Durban, a woman song leader, following an extensive talk on how to make the government to be more proactive in the fight against HIV/AIDS, and how communities must work together to support one another in the fight, intoned "Senzenina?" (What have we done?). "Senzenina" has been noted to be the most prominent song in the antiapartheid struggles besides Enoch Sontonga's "Nkosi Sikelel'iAfrika," to the extent that Duma Ndlovu, the South African screenwriter and activist compared it to "We Shall Overcome" in the American Civil Rights Movement (see Hirsch 2002).

As if in affirmation of Mandela's language preference therefore, the different participants that I have cited appropriated the "struggles" discourse in their interpretations of the HIV/AIDS pandemic. In the domain of musical production, the idea of the *ingoma yomzabalazo* (music of the struggles)[2] is transferred to the context of the "new struggle" with the HIV/AIDS. Thus, in each instance, artists and musicians are implicated in the discursive paradigm thanks to the ways in which they adapt preexisting expressive materials and reinterpreting and infusing them with new meanings in the context of the "new struggle."

ON AIDS MUSIC ETHNOGRAPHY

A number of studies on the culture and politics of health as it relates to HIV/AIDS in particular have been produced since the 1990s. Anthropologists especially have provided the most important frameworks analyzing the phenomenon of HIV/AIDS as cultural issue and as matter of the exercise of social and political power. In 1987, Paula Treichler made an important observation about HIV/AIDS as "an epidemic of signification."[3] Her writing speaks to how social and cultural processes and political dynamics account for the ways in which AIDS has been interpreted and how meanings have been constructed around the disease in local contexts and on the global scene. In line with Treichler's study, some other scholars have read the dynamics in terms of the culture of class differentials, which creates the environment of systemic "structural violence" (see Farmer 2005: 20–40; 1999: 1488), due to social and economic inequalities. For Famer, the cultural politics of classism means that the poor are the most vulnerable and so at risk of the assaults and violations of their rights thanks to the health inequalities in many societies and the refusal to address them.

The theoretical model of cultural signification and power relationships have also shaped the flurry of studies on HIV/AIDS in Africa whereby local forms of cultural constructions of meanings have been interpreted as both inhibitors to, or as resourceful means of awareness intervention for disease prevention (Feldman 2011; Baxen and Breidlid 2009; Jardin 2006; and Booth 2004). Some others have also produced studies that highlight the north-south disparities in economic, cultural, and political power in the context of the African experiences of AIDS (Crane 2013; Sausser 2009; and Rodlach 2006).

The theoretical models have also been channeled in studies on the phenomenon of AIDS in South Africa especially by scholars of public health and social medicine who see the complexity of South Africa's cultural and political history as having serious impact on the current experience of the HIV/AIDS in the country (Karim 2009: 921; Coovadia 2009: 817–34; Fassin 2007: 72; Brummer 2002: 1–26). The history has also shaped the AIDS discourse in South Africa and how the problem is sometimes viewed through the lens of race and ethnicity,[4] thereby fueling a process of cultural politics reminiscent of, and similar to that which characterized apartheid politics and colonialism (Magazinner 2010; de Gruchy and de Gruchy 2005). Hence the discourse on culture and politics of health has also shaped the local constructions of meanings and responses to the AIDS epidemic. Steven Robins, for example, argued that former, president Thabo Mbeki administration's "AIDS denialism" was somewhat of Black nationalist posturing that interpreted the "black disease"[5] labeling of HIV/AIDS and the Medical Science Research Council's statistics of the HIV prevalence in the Black community as another evidence of the continuation of the "long colonial and apartheid legacy of scientific racism" (2004: 651–672). Ultimately the political debates on AIDS fueled suspicions about the scientific studies and reports in Black communities in which many people advanced racialist readings of the disease in ways that are ever more radical (Fassin 2007: 72). In the light of the radical readings, AIDS has also been imagined as "the new apartheid" (McNeill 2011: 2–7), primarily because people infected by HIV are perceived as the victims of misguided public health policies, but also because HIV/AIDS has forced debates about cultural practices with opinions sometimes split along ethnic and racial lines. Thus for instance, the revival of certain cultural practices such as virginity testing among the Zulu as a means to regenerate cultural pride in a post-apartheid South Africa and as local preventive solution to the AIDS crisis generated polarizing debate about its appropriateness (Scorgie 2002: 55). Interestingly in his recent study among the Venda in the Limpopo Province, Fraser McNeill (2011) observed how activists and those who are devoted to grassroots preventive education mobilize similar "traditions" such as girls initiation rites in an attempt to secure legitimacy for their biomedical model. Thus they pitch themselves sometimes against the older women managers of the rites of passage who "invoke authoritative notions of the past to support their stake in resolving the perceived crisis of reproduc[*tive*] *health*" (McNeill 2011: 18). Clearly, Fraser McNeil's work began to shift the conversation and analytical approach. Whereas he channels existing studies that highlight the role of music as culturally based intervention protocols for behavioral change (Steingo 2011: 343–61; Barz and Cohen 2008: 148–159; Barz 2006; DiClemente 1992; and Gottlieb 1990), his study reveals how the domain of musical performance also comprises the sphere of contestations of cultural meaning in the context of HIV and AIDS. Frazer used the songs of female rites of passage and wandering minstrels among the Venda of South Africa to investigate the ways in which biomedical understanding of the human immuno deficiency virus has been rejected in the local understandings of health, illness, sex, and death. In this work, I extend the conversation that McNeil has started by examining a host of other sociocultural and political issues from the perspective of the Siphithemba Choir within the contexts of their actual experiences and musical performances at both local and international levels.

Having been deemed the epicenter of the global AIDS pandemic, a number of studies have also been conducted specifically on South Africa that are focused on AIDS music. Louise Bourgault observes regarding the use of music and other creative and expressive forms that South Africans are "adapting their folkways—recitation, song, dance, dramatic styles, and so on, that had moved them in the past, to the information needs of AIDS prevention" (2003: xxv). "The past" as observed by her is largely the period of the anti-apartheid struggles. Thus, her observation hints at how South Africans have inscribed the struggle against HIV/AIDS into the history of their struggles in general. This is especially evidenced in the 46664 Live Aid Concert, which is a partnership between Rock Star Bono and the Nelson Mandela Children Foundation (See Barz and Cohen 2008: 148–159). As I indicated earlier, I made similar observations of the use of the 46664 symbol in other non-musical contexts, first during the 20-20 Cricket World Cup in South Africa in 2007, and then again as part of billboard anti-AIDS display in Durban in 2012. The current deployments of the apartheid symbols here have double implications. First, by using Nelson Mandela's prison number 46664, the organizers of the Live Aid concert, the activists at the cricket tournament, and the composers of the billboards bring the personality of Nelson Mandela, an embodiment of the antiapartheid struggle, to bear upon the current fight against AIDS as "the new struggle." Secondly, it is illustrative of what the South African musicologists Grant Olwage described as the "non-conclusions and continuations" of the story of apartheid (2008: 8). In the introduction to the collection of essays *Composing Apartheid,* Olwage argued that the end of apartheid may not be construed as the end of the apartheid story, especially because in the ongoing social fallout of apartheid, the present realities, and I dare include the present problem of HIV/AIDS and the larger problem of health inequalities, cannot be ignored (2008: 8).

DEALING WITH THE POLITICS OF ETHNOGRAPHY

After one of the Sunday afternoon choir rehearsals, early in the course of my study with the Siphithemba Choir, Phumlani the choir director asked to ride in my car back to his house, which is just a stone throw from Sizwe's house. He said that he had something for me. Phumlani did not let me into his house, instead he asked me to wait outside while he went into the house. Within seconds, he emerged with some slice of cake unwrapped in a piece of aluminum foil and handed it to me. I thought about wrapping the cake up in the foil and taking it to eat it at home. On a second thought, I decided to cut a piece from the slice, ate it there and then, commented on the tastiness of the cake, and thanked him for the gift. Then I went on to finish the rest of cake since what was left of the slice was too small to pretend to take it home. "For what party?" I thought.

On my way home, I pondered what this gift of tiny piece of cake was all about. By this time in the course of my work with the choir, I was beginning to get into the habit of giving some choir members rides home. Sometimes I dropped off other members in the city so to shorten their travel as well as reduce the cost of transportation for them. On this Sunday, Phumlani literally ordered them to take public transport home because he was going to have a discussion with me. They all obliged to his instructions surprisingly without even offering to wait out this August meeting with me.

None of what happened made immediate sense to me until much later when Phumlani began to frequently refer to me in the meetings as "one of us." The picture also became much clearer as I interacted with other HIV/AIDS support groups too. I came to the realization that a heuristic ethnography of AIDS music entails a complex web of ethnographer–collaborators' relationship. Linda Smith has drawn attention to the fact that research participants can be suspicious of research and researchers, because in the past, these were intertwined with the project of colonization (1999: 3). I knew that this form of distrust for research could be strong, even in a postcolonial, post-apartheid South African society. It proved to be more so in this study because HIV/AIDS has placed extra burdens of social stigma on a large number of Black South Africans, who already live on the margins of the society. While the effects of apartheid still linger in their lives, they are once again made victims from a virus, which has become politicized, nationally and internationally. They are dismayed about being "statisticized," even in a society that emphasizes the humanity of the individual as a member of the community. In addition to this, people living with AIDS are double victims of the virus by virtue of the burden of social stigma associated with the disease.

On my part, I brought with me a baggage of identities that I overlaid on the above scenario: a research scholar from an American university, an African, a Roman Catholic priest, and most of all, one whose human immuno-viral status they did not know, but whose "standard of life" made me appear unaffected by the disease, and therefore by virtue of which I could be suspect. I must confess that each of these identities proved to be of merit and demerit, depending on the spirituality and political consciousness of the persons I was involved with at a given time.

First of all, as a priest, I had to deal with the feeling of betrayal by Christians living with AIDS because they have more often than not been judged, rejected, and let down by their spiritual community, which should have been their bastion of hope. On several occasions, I was confronted by people living with AIDS, caregivers and AIDS counselors, on why the church was still refusing to embrace condom use as a means to check the spread of HIV/AIDS. The issue is that the church, following the directives of Pope Paul VI's encyclical *Humanae Vitae,* considers condom use a form of contraception, which it prohibits; in addition, both the Roman Catholic Church and other conservative religious groups presently have construed condom use as fueling sexual promiscuity. Hence, the shift in emphasis to preaching abstinence. Dick Day describes this as emphasis on the "big A, big B, and little c"[6] (2003: 181). The chief exponents of the big A and big B have largely been the American evangelical groups, with PEPFAR, under former president George W. Bush, as its political bulwark. The irony is that I was also confronted even within the four walls of Roman Catholic AIDS projects. During one of my visits to the St. Clement Catholic Home-Based Care, I had a heated debate with a senior nursing sister. Above the door connecting the makeshift office with the food kitchen hung a sign that read "Use Common Sense not Condom Sense." The sister challenged me on the feasibility of such a doctrine, and after debating the pros and cons of "common sense" versus "condom sense," she reminded me, as I was about to leave for the day, "be sure to keep using common sense and not condom sense."

In a support-group meeting I attended, Zanele (pseudonym) without anything I remember as a cause other than the mention that I am a priest, complained in tears how she had been made to feel guilty as a Catholic because of the church's anti-condom stance. She currently lived with a childhood friend who had walked back into her life after her boyfriend, with whom she has two children, had died of AIDS, about five years before. Zanele was HIV positive, but her children and current partner were negative; or so she believed because she could not say with certainty that her partner had been tested. Her partner cared for her and her two children like a father, even when most of her family members had distanced themselves from her. He had proposed marriage to her, but she was worried about consenting to his proposal. Her greatest concern was that she could not provide satisfaction in a conjugal relationship to a man who loves and cares for her and her children simply because her church prohibited condom use. Meanwhile, she was worried that she could infect him, thereby risking making her children future orphans without the benefit of a father-figure in their lives. At this, I realized that the church had not made room for this type of situation in her position against condom use. All these doctrinal regulations seem to have contributed to the moralization about HIV/AIDS, thus fueling the social stigmatizing of people living with AIDS. Even today, some churches refuse to introduce AIDS programs in their faith communities in the belief that morally responsible children of God cannot contract HIV/AIDS. Thus, as a priest, I embody, to many of the people living with AIDS that I work with, the church and its doctrines and attitudes, which they believe are not compassionate toward them. To such people, I had to present myself as an individual, a student conducting studies not on behalf of the church, but for the benefit of my own knowledge. But most especially, I had to make them understand that my research was designed to help them tell their stories. Kay Shelemay has argued that the ethnographer is a mediator, who intervenes between the community and the outside world, but also to the members of the community by "raising awareness of *their* tradition *and situation*" (1997: 200, italics mine). In doing this, I follow the precedent of Gregory Barz, who writes that:

> faced with the dilemma of representation, I chose to embrace the tool of my trade, ethnography, not only because I can write, but for my own sense of partnership and solidarity with the individuals detailed in this study, I have to write. I only hope that within the inherently flawed medium of academic ethnography that some truth of the lives of those actively engaged in the struggle with AIDS will come through the text. (2006: 2)

By amplifying my position in a research design that I call ethnographic advocacy, I can get the people I study with to look at me differently, trust me, and give me the opportunity to relate with them in a manner that enriches their experience and mine through our encounter. But that did not happen at once. It took several meetings with the groups and one-on-one interactions with individuals such as the "cake meeting" I had with Phumlani, before many of them felt comfortable enough with me to open up and tell me their stories. Once they felt comfortable enough with me, they revealed that as people living with AIDS, they are weary of being judged. Their suspicion was not only limited to churchmen like me, but even to lay people who happen to be HIV-negative—until a time they were convinced that they were open and honest, and not morally biased against them.

In addition to the scenarios outlined above, there is the question of insider–outsider perspective. A pertinent issue is whether an African studying another African community makes me a cultural insider or outsider. My first reaction to this is if the status of insider is determined by geographical nativity or race, then perhaps I could be considered an insider. But this position is hardly tenable with respect to this study, for the following reason: while in South Africa, I heard people refer to me on several occasions as *ikwerekwere*. This word (plural, *amakwerekwere*) means 'stranger,' and is used to categorize all non-Zulu and, by extension, all non-South Africans who sojourn in the country, particularly in search of greener pastures. I never heard this term being used for people of European origin and Asians, not even those who had relocated to South Africa in recent years from North America, the U.K., Eastern Europe, the Scandinavian countries, and South Asia. The term was used more exclusively for people from Africa north of the Limpopo. *Amakwerekwere* has a negative and arguably violent connotation. The evidence of this is the unprecedented violent xenophobic attacks on African immigrants in some of the major cities of South Africa in 2008, 2009, 2010, 2012, and 2013. They were accused of usurping their hard-won opportunities in terms of housing and jobs (see www.csvr.org.za).

I will confess that each time I mentioned that I was coming from the United States, I could feel some sense of relief with people, and more welcoming attitudes. But then that created another layer of a problematic relationship. As Nhlakanipho Gumede, coordinator of the Clermont Community Resource Center based at the St. Clement Catholic Mission, told me in his office, upon my first meeting with him, "these days a lot of us, especially members of our support groups [who are all HIV+] are worried that people are always coming from overseas to study us, collect information about us, and then go home leaving us the way we are." In this conversation, he expressed hope that I must be coming with a different attitude, being an African who by default must share their sensibilities as people who have been oppressed. Even some members of Siphithemba sometimes voiced concern about being used as exhibitions in medical science communities in North America to make the case for funding HIV/AIDS research. This is notwithstanding that they value the opportunity to travel to America and the United Kingdom for performances. According to Phumlani, I am the first African to work with them, and the first to be primarily interested in their music, more than in the fact that they are HIV-positive people. These remarks bear a tone of ambivalence. One could assume that, as an African, I am a cultural insider, yet the tone of disquietude about being a research scholar from an American university casts me in the shadow of those who have come before me. This ambivalent form of relationship is what I call the *insider–outsider position* in a culture community of research. This is because the meaning associated with "research" evokes the imbalance of power in "colonial" environment as Linda Smith noted, saddled with a feeling of paranoia and insecurity that is similar to what Franz Fanon described as the "nervous condition of the native" (1967). This does not mean, however, that I was always treated like an outsider in all instances.

Lila Abu-Lughod (1993) alludes to issues related to her identity and how this played out in the course of her fieldwork with Bedouin women of Egypt. She explicitly acknowledged her multiple identities, which had a bearing upon how she was received in the community. Whether it was her ethnic identity as a "halfie,"[7] or as an unmarried woman, and a married woman without a child, or even as a social role model (1993: 38), her identity had an impact on the nature of the intersubjectivity she had with the people she was studying. In a like manner, my multiple identities as American student on a research mission, and as a Black African from Nigeria, shaped how the people I worked with related with me. There were certainly moments when I was an outsider, and moments when I felt like an insider. Those moments when I conversed extensively with them in IsiZulu, those moments when I would remove my shirt and join in the broiling of meat or even drink *utshwala* (a local brew, made from millet) with them, those moments when I joined in conversations that revisited the impacts of colonialism and apartheid, those moments when I tended to agree with them that their ANC-led government had not done enough to curb the spread of HIV/AIDS and comparing that with the corrupt and reckless government of Nigeria—such moments saw me being treated like one of them. Knowing about my multiple identities compelled me to undergo a form of self-ethnography (Latta 1999), by which I interrogate the nature of my research and what I write about. I see my work as an exploration of South African choral music, as narratological material, with which I critique the artistic confrontation with HIV/AIDS, whose effects have conspired with the mistakes of the post-apartheid government to prolong the structure of hegemonic feelings that are heard in their songs.

Overall, I believe that the multiple identities were beneficial to the final outcome of this study. As a priest, I had easy access to religious institutions such as the Diakonia Council of Churches and the Pietermaritzburg Agency for Christian Social Awareness, and to some religious leaders and theologians, from whom I garnered insight into the work of their institutions. Many support groups and individuals felt very at home with me because they believed that I shared their cultural sensibilities as an African. But that is as long as cultural sensibility was concerned. Sometimes, being an African—and more so, a Nigerian—constituted initial obstacles to access to certain groups; however, the idea that I was an American, from an academic institution, often brought some sense of relief to individuals.

My multiple identities were further compounded with regard to the Siphithemba Choir and other HIV/AIDS support groups with which I worked, precisely because of the problem of stigma. However, by sharing meals with them, visiting individual members in their homes, and offering to take individuals out for lunch and dinner on their birthdays, I helped dispel doubts they may have had about me as someone who might be judgmental toward them. Their feeling at home with me meant that I could assess information easily whenever I had the need. Yet my status as a priest modified the nature of my relationship with them, both as a group and as individuals. The Catholics and non-Catholics among them sometimes called me by my name, and at other times they called me *umfundisi* 'priest' or "Father Austin." That way of referencing meant that I was consciously treated as a priest sometimes. I cannot ascertain how much information may have been withheld from me on account of my priestly status and the expectation that I maintain a certain level of distance. I know however, that I was privileged by virtue of my priestly status, to gain information from individual members about their personal lives and experience with their HIV status, in a manner that is similar to that of the confessional and spiritual direction, otherwise called *internal forum* in Roman Catholic pastoral practice. For this reason, I found my role constantly shifting between that of a researcher and that of a priest. I treaded on a fine line all the time; and as I write this work, I have to make conscious decisions about what I must or must not include as ethnographic data. I cannot, however, argue that some of the information I gained from the *internal forum* has not affected my interpretations of issues hereof, but I have been careful to separate and to keep such data out of this work.

As an African Catholic priest from America engaged in fieldwork in Africa, I am struck by the complexity of my relationship with the Siphithemba Choir and other individuals and groups I worked with in this research. While seeking to balance my cultural insider–outsider role in this research, as has been advocated by ethnomusicologists (Burnim 1985b), I had the extra burden of balancing my spiritual and temporal role in my relationship with my collaborators. This was not an easy task, but what helped me was the realization that my research was primarily to help my collaborators tell the story of their experience of HIV/AIDS within the complexity of their own social, political, and economic history.

FRAMEWORK AND LAYERS OF ANALYSIS

In the light of theoretical models that have been propounded by anthropologists and sociologists, and scholars of AIDS music, I wish to lay out hereby the various levels at which I analyze the Siphithemba Choir and their music. First I situate my discourse against the backdrop of the social and economic environment that fuels the spread of HIV/AIDS in South Africa. The poverty and loss of traditional family structure and cultural values because of the apartheid-era migrant-labor system are being confronted in the organization of the choral-music ensemble, which now brings economic empowerment and a strongly cohesive social structure and support system for members of the choir. Such use of music has precedence in African examples. Christopher A. Waterman's (1990) study of *jùjú* among the Yoruba of Nigeria reveals that music plays the role of wealth redistribution in an economically asymmetrical society. In a similar vein, Ruth M. Stone (2008) discusses how the Woni Group (Moses Woni and John Woni) took advantage of money that flowed into Liberian rubber camps on paydays by relying on patrons who sponsored their performances on such dates at the rubber estates. On the social level, such organization and performance of music creates a process and environment for negotiating group identity for members who share a common experience of being HIV-positive. Within such an environment, music is communally created, mirroring the message of hope in the possibility of overcoming the disease through collective effort. Hence, I posit that the study of the use of music must look beyond the communicative value of music, and must include the organization of music as a social process.

Relying upon issues articulated in their music vis-à-vis the discursive linking of the AIDS and apartheid, I study the Siphithemba Choir and its music as a form of struggle and resistance, which mirrors Black South Africans' experience of struggle on different levels, and their act of struggle and resistance is staged on several fronts at the same time. For this reason also, my analyses of the choir and their performances participate on several levels. First is the choir members' use of their musical performance to resist the virus, which is directly responsible for their social and economic estrangement in a system in which the circumstance of history and human politics has conspired and already contributed to placing them on the margins of society. The second level is the members' resistance to the cultural maxims that contribute to their being stigmatized and discriminated as bearers of disease that is inimical to their communities. On a third level, is the apartheid element that crept into the AIDS discourse in South Africa, when activists began to refer to the disease and the circumstances of government's ineffectual response to the epidemic as "the new apartheid" (Rivière 2002; Gevisser 2001). For the Siphithemba Choir members however, AIDS as "the new apartheid" consists also in politics of culture, dynamics of inter-racial relationships that impinge upon the public perceptions of the disease in a "post-apartheid" environment, as well as other aspects of the global politics of AIDS, including the issue of patent rights on the ARV that is exerted by the Western pharmaceutical giants. And finally is the politics of representation that characterize the choir's relationship with the scientific community with who the choir members collaborate in the CD4/Viral Load and antiretroviral researches. As I will show in this work, the political nature of this relationship hinges on the question of whose voice is more important—the scientists whose story purport to subsume the choir's stories in their eagerness to showcase the choir and members' vibrant singing and dancing as evidence of success in scientific endeavors, or the choir members who tell the story of their experience of the disease through their music and dance, and whose ingenuous use of music preceded their collaboration with the scientists.

Siphithemba's music as struggle and resistance can however be fully grasped when placed in the context of Black South African, and indeed Zulu historical uses of music as struggle. To do this, I take a multi-pronged approach that juxtaposes the choir's use of music in the context of HIV and AIDS with the use of music in different historical moments including apartheid, and previous instances of disease outbreaks of epidemiological magnitude. My use of historical framework here tallies with the increasing call for historiography in the field of ethnomusicology, especially since Tim Rice advocated in 1987 for a historiographical model that analyzes the "formative processes" in and of music as cultural production (473). About a decade later, Virginia Danielson offered a more insightful case study of the importance of historical research when she historically situated Umm Kulthūm within the larger context of Egyptians' public conversation on music and social life by relying extensively on archival resources. The value of such an approach in her study lies in her ability to make "comparison of interpretations of events as they occurred with later reflections on similar events and offer a view of the usages of events from the past to illustrate larger ideas or trends and to explain or shape the present" (1997: 7). By this means, Danielson ultimately answered her basic question about why Umm Kulthūm among so many other entertainers is so important, and why and how she could sustain her popularity for so long (1997: 2). By following similar path in my study of the Siphithemba Choir, I hope to demonstrate the historical significance of this choral ensemble on two important levels. First, the ideas articulated in their music and the social processes that undergird their musical activities are rooted in, draw upon, as well as mirror historical antecedents of musical activities in Black South African (and Zulu) experiences of wars, conflicts, and struggles that have become integral to their sense of nationhood and cultural identity. This is to the extent in which HIV/AIDS became a factor in re-enacting and sustaining the interracial (and inter-class) acrimonious relationships that speak to the issues of power dynamics that is by the way "culturally constructed" through "knowledge making, universe construction, and the social production of feeling and of 'reality' through discourses" (Averill 1997: 1). The second follows from the first. The tapestry of ideas articulated in the choir's music and their organizing is diagnostic of a desire to inscribe themselves as social, economic, political and cultural agents with the disposition to monitor the domains, and to negotiate the flow of human intersubjective interactions (Giddens 1984: 30), so that they act as human subjects who participate in the social maintenance of the historically generated knowledge making and universe construction of their community, which now impinge upon their perceptions and interpretations of the HIV/AIDS pandemic.

By focusing on the Siphithemba Choir as case study, this research reveals a convergence of three streams of activity in the struggle with HIV/AIDS. First, as a choral ensemble that originated in a mission institution where it functioned as a community-based HIV/AIDS support group and income-generating project, Siphithemba exemplifies the transformation of an approach previously used in the antiapartheid struggles by creating community-based self-help income projects. Second, members of the Siphithemba Choir perceive that since Black people in South Africa and on the continent of Africa comprise the majority of the victims of HIV/AIDS, the choir should position itself as an advocate for the African cause. Events related to contestation over cultural symbols, such as the use of Zulu drums (discussed in chapter 7), recalls the politics of culture that characterized the forms of power contestation in mission Christianity and under apartheid. These issues therefore connect them to the earlier use of choral singing in the mission church as a form of resistance that was occasioned by the experience of discrimination. Similarly, like some Black eclectic composers in the past, they deploy their singing as a means to articulate and address this experience in the context of the HIV/AIDS discourse.

Finally, these issues are interspersed on different levels of analyses, namely the McCord Hospital, (South) Africa, and the worldwide stage, according to where they are played out and with what degree of significance. It is my hope that by the end, I shall have successfully presented a multilayered stream of narrative about the Siphithemba Choir, in respect to how they perform their experience of the HIV/AIDS.

ETHNOGRAPHIC STYLE AND STRUCTURE OF WORK

The anecdotal and narratological style with which this introductory chapter was opened is a pointer to the strong leaning in phenomenological writing in this work. It will be disingenuous of me to assume that my reader would naturally accept that my research collaborators thought through some of the issues that I raise and analyze in this work and then handed them over to me in the course of my research. By introducing the major issues addressed in the various chapters of this book using stories of real events and activities, and then analytically situating them in the larger context of the HIV/AIDS discourse, my aim is to show how I know what I know. By so doing I join in the league of ethnomusicologists and sociocultural anthropologists who have found value in reflexive writing (see Jackson 1989; Abu-Lughod 1993; Kisliuk 1998; Reed 2003). Theirs are in furtherance of the model of sociological phenomenology of Alfred Schultz (1967), whose logic of the "life world" explains the social nature of knowledge wherein meaning is generated in social reality via the dynamics of intersubjectivity.

On another level, the phenomenological style affords the ethnographer the benefit of reflective intermission between the time in which the event is experienced and the actual writing; that is, "meaning is created when *durée*[8] is broken by reflection by looking back on earlier experience" (Stone 2008: 166). For me' I had the benefit of engaging in reflective writings at different moments during my field trips and upon return from the field. I identified a number of emergent issues about which I would make follow-ups so that I engaged my collaborators in more in-depth scrutiny in order to understand what it is they are thinking about, and how their thoughts may have informed the ways in which they chose to articulate their experiences of HIV and AIDS, the meanings they make of their experiences, and how those find expression in their organizational activities and musical production. The further implication in this writing approach is that it let me move away from the "objectivist" worldview (Johnson 1987: xxxvii), a paradigm that has characterized anthropological and social-science research since the late nineteenth century, to letting the data—the music and music events and participants' interpretations of their activities—inform my analyses. The objectivist worldview subscribes to the purported sense of neutrality, albeit what Linda T. Smith (1999: 55–56) calls "distancing" in research. Yet "distancing" or "neutrality" is not without colonial burdens, especially as researchers rely on Western-derived theoretical frameworks for analyses of the cultural behaviors of the peoples they study. Under such "bird's-eye perspective" ethnography (Erlmann 1996: 11), in the Western episteme has constituted the "rules by which *the world of our participants* has been theorized [and analyzed, and therefore] *their* voices have been overwhelmingly silenced" (Smith 1999: 29). While the reflexive writing lets my collaborators, their music and their extramusical signifiers speak for themselves, I do so knowing that my personal experience in my involvement with the choir comprise the lens through which I engage and analyze the issues that are articulated in their music.

I have organized the chapters of this book in a manner that I believe holds them together. Together the chapters address different aspects of the issues that have been raised in this introductory chapter, which I have used to set the stage for appreciating how the AIDS discourse and the politics of the disease is articulated in the music of the Siphithemba Choir. Chapters 2 and 3 are historical in nature; chapter 2 discourses the history of the founding of the Siphithemba Choir at McCord Hospital in Durban, their growth and contribution to the Sinikthemba AIDS clinic and the general AIDS program which has been recognized as the first of its kind in Africa. The story is also situated within the larger history and mission of the hospital whose holistic approach to caring for the sick, integrated with sociocultural activities such as the nurses and staff choir, preceded the Siphithemba Choir as a music ensemble and HIV/AIDS support group of individuals who receive spiritual counseling and benefit from the clinical care of the sick. Chapter 3 investigates the historical musical responses to disease epidemics such as smallpox, which plagued the region for more than two centuries between 1713 and early 1900s, and the 1918 influenza. By juxtaposing case studies of musical responses to historical smallpox and influenza epidemics with the current use of music in the HIV/AIDS experience, the chapter explores the meanings that people make of their experiences of epidemics. Through a close reading of the song examples, I suggest that sociocultural factors such as race and ethnicity, economics, and spirituality comprise important frameworks for constructing meanings around the issue of health and in the context of epidemics, thus informing some of the dynamics in the current discourses of AIDS and public health realities in present-day South Africa, and how those dynamics manifest in the music of the Siphithemba choir.

Returning to the Siphithemba Choir proper, chapter 4 examines the way in which the group functions as a community of mutual support, and how the indigenous Nguni *Ubuntu* philosophy is used to foster their sense of community and mutual well-being, as well as re-validate themselves as productive members of society. In chapters 5 and 6, I return to the music of the Siphithemba Choir proper. Chapter 5 examines the style of music that the choir performs, and how their songs reflect their spirituality. Grouping their songs thematically allows the reader to appreciate their sociocultural perspectives, the historical and cultural roots of the perspectives, and how they might explain the choir members, experience of HIV/AIDS and their interpretations of those experiences. In chapter 6, I explore the processes of their musical production, which demonstrate how their sense of community also translates into their communal approach to musical composition, performance, and as expression of community ethos.

Chapters 7 and 8 examine different aspects of the sociopolitical dynamics that participate in the AIDS discourse and how the Siphithemba Choir engages these issues in and through their music. Chapter 7 addresses the issue of politics of culture in the context of AIDS using the example of the controversy over the use of the *idlamu* drum steeped in contestations of cultural meanings and spirituality between the choir and the White superintendent of McCord Hospital. It examines the politics of racial identity, that big elephant in the room that often seem to be sidestepped by anthropologists and ethnomusicologists who engage in the ethnography of AIDS and AIDS music. In chapter 8, I shift to a different kind of politics, namely the dynamics of relationship between the choir and the scientific community with whom they collaborate in the research for AIDS treatment. I argue that the research scientists by virtue of their position wield a lot of power that allows them to control the conversation to the extent of subsuming the story of the choir under the scientists' story as experts on the AIDS epidemic. Unbeknown to them however, the choir figured out ways to use their songs and the concert stage to subvert the power of the scientists and establish their voices as better advocates on their behalf and on behalf of all Africans who suffer the debilitating effects of the virus. In the concluding chapter, I return to the national and global politics of health and reflect on how Siphithemba's music engages these politics and the implications of my approach to analyzing the choir and their music through the lens of racial, cultural, and global politics.

On a final note, the name Siphithemba is used by the choir currently, but the group went by the name Sinikithemba at its initial founding, named after the Sinikthemba Clinic (the HIV/AIDS clinic at McCord Hospital) and the support group that gave rise to the choir. Hence in this work, I will use Siphithemba to always refer to the choir, and Sinikithemba to refer to the clinic and the support group whenever applicable.

NOTES

1. For more on the policies and controversies, see Nattrass (2007).
2. See Lee Hirsch. (2002). *Amandla! A revolution in four-part harmony,* for a more extant reference to the antiapartheid music production as *ingoma yomzabalazo* by the famous South African voice diva Sibongile Khumalo.
3. See also Treichler Paula A. (2004). *How to Have Theory in an Epidemic.* Durham, NC: Duke University Press.
4. See Okigbo,"Performing Blackness in a South African HIV/AIDS Choir." *Du Bois Review* 8, no. 1 (2011). In this article, I argued that the Siphithemba Choir's performance of Blackness is shaped by a combination of several related factors, namely the nature of the virus's genome and its racial and geographical distribution, the history of apartheid and its lingering effects, the interracial acrimony in the post-apartheid society, and other sociocultural and global politics of HIV and AIDS.
5. See also Karim who observed that "black disease" labeling was actually framed by the apartheid government in the 1980s just to reinforce racial prejudices about Black sexual promiscuity (Karim et al., 2009: 923).
6. ABC is the acronym of a widespread African slogan, "Abstinence, Be Faithful, Condomize."
7. The word is a colloquial one, used to describe her double ethnic or national identity: Arab and American.
8. Durée is the "qualitative or inner time that is distinct from quantitative or outer time" (see Stone 2008: 166).

Chapter 2

The Making of the Siphithemba Choir

On Tuesday, August 7, 2007, I met with Dr. Helga Holst, the medical superintendent at McCord Hospital in Durban. As a middle-aged White woman, Dr. Holst presided over what was reckoned as one of the best "holistic HIV [and AIDS] care" in Africa[1] under which program the Siphithemba Choir was born. Our meeting lasted a little over an hour, during which the superintendent recounted the history of the choir, placing it in the context of the story of the hospital as a church institution. She rehashed the story of Dr. McCord, the American Congregationalist and medical missionary whose work and vision gave birth to a hospital that would later be named after him. According Dr. Holst, the story of McCord Hospital is in tandem with the work that goes on at the institution as a health-care asset, but also as a spiritual healing center for those afflicted by illness. According to her,

> here we are dedicated to providing physical, spiritual, and emotional care for the sick and the people around them in their families. When we formed the HIV/AIDS support group for instance, we hoped that we could serve both those who are infected, as well as those who are affected, that is their immediate families. So this place is for the practice of medicine, but it is also a place of prayer and spiritual activities.

I wanted to visit the hospital chapel, so I inquired of her about the location of the chapel, to which she responded, "The entire hospital is a sanctuary." It took some seconds for the meaning of that assertion to sink in, but it made more sense when in the course of my research I realized how much presence the resident chaplain has in the entire facility.

Dr. Helga Holst's narrative on the history of the hospital also explains that the Siphithemba Choir is more than just a group of individuals engaged in the fight against the HIV and AIDS within the space of McCord Hospital. Its story is also representative of Black South Africans' experience of the colonial encounters, and the merits of mission Christianity among Africans especially in the area of public health. Through a narrative of the story of the choir's founding at McCord Hospital, I suggest that the space of the mission hospital was a fertile ground for the birth of such a creative approach to the fight against HIV and AIDS, using the tool of music that expresses faith and hope.

MCCORD HOSPITAL: A HEALTH MISSION TO THE ZULU

The missionary project in Africa has been construed as part of the colonial project on the continent, but Christian missionaries are known to have brought with them, as part of their evangelization and pastoral efforts, health-care systems that helped local communities cope with diseases that indigenous health practices hitherto had not treated effectively. Today, the health-care infrastructure in sub-Saharan Africa is still largely that erected by missionaries and faith-based institutions, both during colonialism and in the postcolonial periods (ARHAP 2006: 121).

In southern Africa, the earliest educational and health institutions, built by English and Dutch missionaries, catered to the settler communities. Roman Catholic and American missionaries were latecomers in the region. By 1825, the American Board of Commissioners for Foreign Missions of the Presbyterians and Congregationalists from Boston had begun to make inroads, establishing the American Zulu Mission in Natal (Etherington 1997: 89–106). Like their European counterparts, American missionaries established mission schools, most notably the Adams College at the Adams Mission in Amanzintoti, Natal. Dr. McCord, the medical missionary who established the clinic known today as McCord Hospital in Durban in 1909, followed the trail of the American Zulu Mission. The clinic was located first at the Adams Mission in Amanzintoti, but moved to the high point in Durban, where it was transformed into a medical center. Unlike most academic and health institutions in the colony at the time, Dr. McCord's clinic provided services to Europeans and Africans alike, but primarily to the Zulu (McCord 2000: 150). In short, McCord's case is typical of missionary projects that construed mission in sub-Saharan Africa as healing (Allwood 1989: 123–124) and used medical services as a proselytizing tool. In doing this, missionaries like McCord probably understood the dangers inherent in the Cartesian mind–body dualism, which of course has a theological antecedence in the Plato-Philo-Augustinian synthesis in the medieval church. At the heart of the medical missionaries' initiative is the understanding that humans are saved in body and soul. In the words of the theologian James Cochrane, "A church that takes preferential option for the health of the [person] is a church faithful to the healing and wholeness implied by the Latin word *salus,* from which we derive 'salvation' (2006: 18).

Medical services were used to minister to the health needs of converts in the economy of their well-being. In this practice, health-care for the bodily welfare of converts was often paired with the spiritual care of the sick. It is arguable that the success of this approach of evangelization is partly due to the African cosmology of locating health and well-being in religion and its rituals—a cosmology that permeates the rhythms of everyday life (ARHAP 2006).

Accounts of the history of the medical center under Dr. McCord show three important operational components: diagnosis and dispensing of medicines, pastoral (spiritual) care of the sick, and home visitation of the sick (McCord 2000). The second component is of significance in understanding the historical context of the Sinikithemba Clinic and the Siphithemba Choir.

Margaret McCord's documentation showed that Mr. William Makanya, a Black pastor, conducted prayer services with patients at the medical center as early as 1911 (McCord 2000: viii). The practice of retaining a pastor to minister to the spiritual welfare of the sick has continued at the hospital. At the time of the research for this work, Pastor Chili served as the pastoral counselor; playing an important role as spiritual counselor among the members of the HIV/AIDS support group at the Sinikithemba AIDS clinic.

MCCORD HOSPITAL IN THE HISTORY OF EPIDEMICS IN NATAL

McCord Hospital has provided health services for people in Durban and its environs since its inception. Dr. Helga Holst, the hospital's superintendent, says, "the strength of the clinic probably lies in its role in helping the citizens cope with different outbreaks of epidemics in South African history." The current wave of HIV/AIDS and tuberculosis in KwaZulu-Natal has been estimated to be above the level of epidemics, with HIV/AIDS prevalence being above 30 percent in the population of the province. McCord Hospital set the pace in providing treatment and support services to HIV-infected persons. The hospital estimated that at least 50 percent of its medical admissions between 2007 and 2011 are HIV related. That number was up to 70 percent between 1996 and 2007; but this is not new at the hospital.

Margaret McCord's chronicle reveals that Dr. McCord's dispensary provided the largest services to local Zulu communities during the 1904 and 1917–1918 malaria and influenza epidemics, respectively. These epidemics may have seemed then as devastating as the HIV/AIDS pandemic seems now.

Accounts of the earlier epidemics show that they spared no racial, class, or cultural group. Entire families succumbed to the disease, and communities lost important leaders, yet in Natal, Dr. McCord's clinic proved a bastion of hope in the form of treatment and spiritual support to those who were dying or who had lost their loved ones. It is in the light of this history that the significance of the establishment of the Sinikithemba AIDS clinic and support group at McCord Hospital in 1997 becomes evident.

HIV/AIDS: A NEW EPIDEMIC, AND THE BIRTH OF THE SINIKITHEMBA SUPPORT GROUP

In 1997, the antiretroviral cocktail therapy had not yet begun to be widely distributed, at least not in sub-Saharan Africa, but the HIV/AIDS situation in South Africa was already becoming alarming. By then, most medical admissions at McCord hospital were HIV-related. In the absence of significant medical help, HIV-positive persons bore the burden of being stigmatized for their status. The leaders of McCord Hospital, however, understood that alternative help in the form of spiritual counseling and social support system could be useful in helping people cope with the emotional and material burdens associated with being HIV-positive.

Mrs. Nonhlanhla Mhlongo founded the Sinikithemba Support Group and its choral ensemble in 1997. She had trained as a social worker at the University of Zululand between 1975 and 1980. The university was one of the major centers of the South African Students' Organization, the platform for propagating the Black Consciousness Movement, led by Steve Biko. Through her training as a social worker at this university, and her experience of this movement, she followed the philosophy of self-reliance, grassroots networking, and support system as critical forms of intervention in struggle experience—a philosophy at the core of the movement and its allied religious belief, known as Black Theology.

Like most urban Black educated young men and women, Mrs. Mhlongo testified to her love of music: "Even myself, I love singing. I used to sing in the school choir and in the church choirs. I used to even perform solo in the choir [in church and school]." After graduating from college, she worked for the state in the Department of Population and Development, where for sixteen years she put to intense use her skill of working with communities in hands-on field experience.

All these experiences would come to bear on her motivation and success in founding the Sinikithemba Support Group and eventually the choir. At McCord Hospital, her primary responsibility was to coordinate the medical social services and to administer pre- and post-HIV/AIDS-diagnosis counseling.

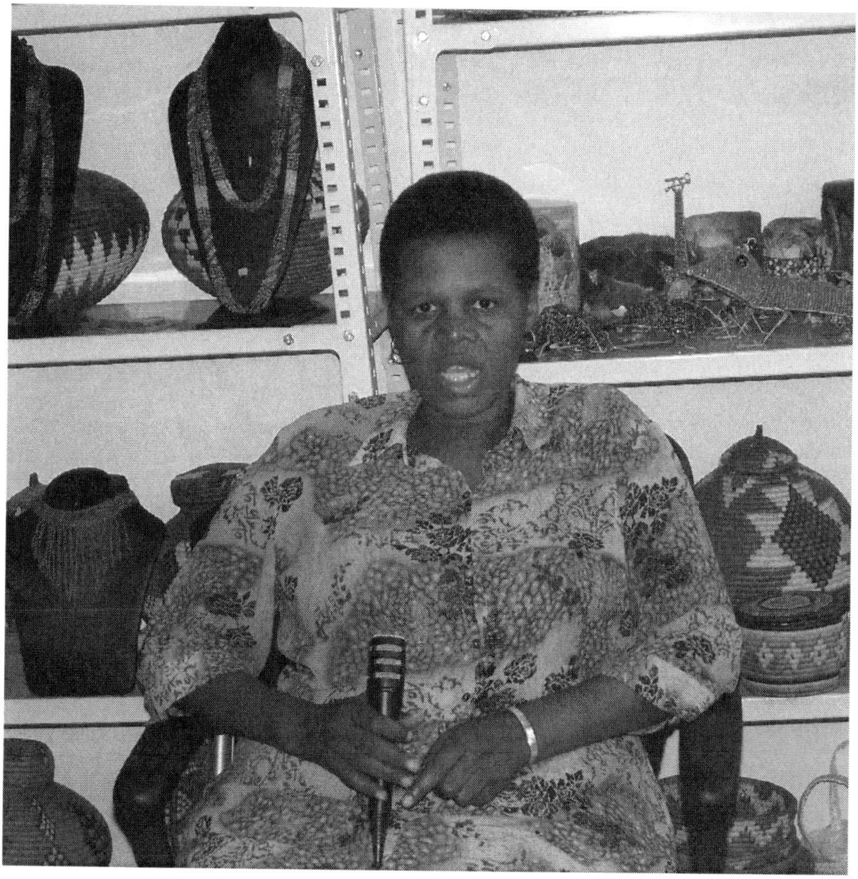

Figure 2.1 Nohlanhla Mhlongo.

The tradition of maintaining the spiritual component of health management in mission health institutions was still in place by the time Mrs. Mhlongo arrived at McCord Hospital, but there is no indication that particular attention was paid to HIV/AIDS patients. In fact, a pastoral counselor and at least two social workers were employed there. The hospital was carrying out a lot of HIV testing, but there was no follow-up mechanism to ensure that those who tested positive returned for counseling and prophylactic care. The problem appeared to have been partly due to the poverty of the patients. Mhlongo described her experience when she arrived at the hospital, patients who came to HIV testing never returned to collect their results, and to follow up with prophylactic treatment if they were positive so their health wouldn't deteriorate. The prevalent excuses were lack of things as basic as food to talk of bus fare. According to her, many of the patients when they returned to the hospital at all, "they will come back on [*sic*] wheel chairs."

According to Mrs. Mhlongo, at some point "a husband and wife were found rotting alive in a township." Apparently, their families and neighbors had abandoned the couple, who were too weak to care for themselves. Later on, Mrs. Mhlongo discovered from the hospital records that the couple had been to McCord for testing, but had not returned for treatment. Her first step in the effort to curb such cases was to use the hospital records to locate patients who had made recent visits to the hospital and to invite them for a special encounter session, during which she would try to persuade them of the need to join the support group.[2]

The group met once a week, on Tuesdays, when its members prayed together and sang hymns and gospel songs. The meetings marked the first instance when members began to gain consciousness of themselves as a singing group. Also, they did Bible reading and "faith sharing," when members narrated their experiences of being HIV-positive, how they were perceived in their families and local communities, how they were coping with the burdens of stigma and rejection, and what strategies they were using to overcome their emotional burdens. According to Mrs. Mhlongo, the initial membership of the support group was about twenty. Records provided by Monty Thomas, the coordinator of the team of AIDS counselors at the clinic at the beginning of this study, show that the support group had roughly five hundred members in its register by the year 2000.

Pastor Sizwe Chili maintained her post at the hospital as spiritual counselor, but she now worked closely with Mrs. Mhlongo to manage the spiritual welfare of the HIV/AIDS Support Group. The pastor conducted prayers for the group and led them in devotions. Occasionally, pastors from other neighboring local churches, particularly the pastor of the United Church of Christ, a bona fide member of the American Congregationalists, were brought in to conduct prayers and devotions and to give words of exhortation to the support group. The practice of bringing in pastors from local churches to conduct prayers and devotions for the group became resourceful in another way: since many of the group's members lacked income and had deficient nutritional habits, some pastors appealed to their faith communities for food, milk, fruits, and vegetables to be distributed to the group during its weekly meetings. In this way, many got relief in their nutrition, while the food distribution served as incentive for others to join the group.

Once the hospital management had approved the forming of the support group, the next move was to give the group a name. Group members thought of a name, and a consensus was reached to adopt the name *Sinikithemba Support Group*. (The word *sinikithemba* in Zulu means 'we give hope' or 'give us hope.') The group's meetings took place at a building in the hospital originally known as House 35 (numbers designate all buildings at McCord), which was soon renamed "Hope House because of the HIV/AIDS thing that was ongoing in the building, and the hope it brought to all people [living with HIV and AIDS] who visited the house" (interview wirh Nomusa Mpanza). Thus, evidently, the location of the group at Hope House influenced the choice of its name, but also, the name indicates the spirituality of hope, which has guided the operation of the hospital since its inception. For those living with HIV and AIDS, the support group and the hospital have been a source of hope and a space where they nurtured their faith, and thus their determination to live. Hope House was also called Sinikithemba Clinic because of the HIV/AIDS clinic that operated in the same building, and the clinic was named after the support group. When the current Sinikithemba AIDS Clinic building was completed, however, the entire HIV/AIDS project was moved to the new building, but House 35 continued to be designated Hope House.

Taking a vernacular name that mirrors the vision of a group is a practice that found strong emphasis especially since the era of the Steve Biko-led Black Consciousness. In 1973, in Kingwilliamstown in the Eastern Cape, Biko started the Black Community Projects, an umbrella of small projects that took Zulu or Xhosa names. The most famous among them was the Zanempilo (We Give Health or We Have Health) Community Health Clinic (founded in 1974), which provided "grass-roots essential health services independent of the government" (Stubbs 2006: 190). The Njwaxa Home Industry was a skill-acquisition center. Today, most groups running similar projects have followed the example of the Black Consciousness Movement in naming their projects. In the course of this fieldwork, I encountered several similar projects. One was the Siyaphila (We Live Well) Project, a community-based HIV/AIDS project in Pietermaritzburg, partly funded by the South African Catholic Bishops. Another was the Nkosinathi (God Is with Us) Project, located at the Emmanuel Cathedral in Durban, where I worked as visiting associate pastor during my stay in Durban; this project runs a HIV/AIDS program plus care for the homeless. At the Sinikithemba Support Group, *hope* was the watchword for all activities. As I show later, "hope" has been a dominant concept and a theme in the choir's songs, and it characterizes the spirituality of the support group and the choir.

By sharing experiences and encouraging one another in words that speak of hope and faith, the sense of family became the guiding force in the inner operations of the support group. According to Mrs. Mhlongo, the group "was like a family. They were supposed to come only on Tuesdays, but people will come on Monday to Friday because of family environment. . . . If a member doesn't show up, Siphokazi [pseudonym], you will see her, she will say 'Where is so and so?'"

With time, the group assumed the responsibility of attending the funerals of deceased members and providing support to bereaved families. When members were sick, other members from their area would go in small numbers to visit and to encourage them. According to Mrs. Mhlongo, the group even collected money to support the children of diseased members. Thus, at this stage, the level of consciousness about the struggle with AIDS has already gone beyond individual experience to a communal one, wherein HIV/AIDS is no longer confronted as just a sickness that affects the individual body, but as a disease that affects the community.

FROM SUPPORT GROUP TO COMMUNITY MICROECONOMIC PROJECT

One of the burdens of the stigma of HIV/AIDS is that many infected persons lost their jobs. Zinhle, a member of the Siphithemba Choir, talks about how she lost her job when a fellow employee accessed her office cabinet without her permission, read her diagnosis result, and revealed her status to her employers, who immediately fired her (Hainsworth 2006). In fact, a majority of members of the support group had never been gainfully employed, some for lack of skills. The lack of a strong financial base resulted in deficient nutritional habits, and these, in turn, resulted in opportunistic infections, such as tuberculosis, pneumonia, and meningitis. For Mrs. Mhlongo, however, this did not have to be so. She believed that while HIV-positive persons are still strong, they could be productive, and should be able to earn a living. She used the support-group meetings to encourage members on the need to look inward and figure out any talents or skills they might have that might benefit their economic conditions. According to her, "We've got people who are HIV-positive, and who have no income. . . . What we are trying to inculcate to people is that they have to work and not beg. Because of their status, they shouldn't go around begging; instead they should give something in return."

It was during one such meeting that an older member who had skill in beadwork offered to teach others how to make beads so as to preoccupy members during their gatherings, with the idea that they could earn money from the effort. This woman used to make and market beads to tourists by the beaches of Durban, but her health had deteriorated, and she developed severe arthritic pain, which made it difficult for her to handle the beading tools and needles. Mrs. Mhlongo provided for the initial project with about R300.00 (roughly US$40.00 at the time when the Rand was exchanging at about R7.00 to US$1.00) by purchasing the required materials. In a short time, the beadwork grew into a major skill-acquisition project, from whose proceeds members achieved gainful employment. The parking lot of Hope House was provided as a space to train members in beadwork, sewing, and knitting. Staff of a local art program were brought in to teach support-group members how to make mosaics (see figure 2.2).

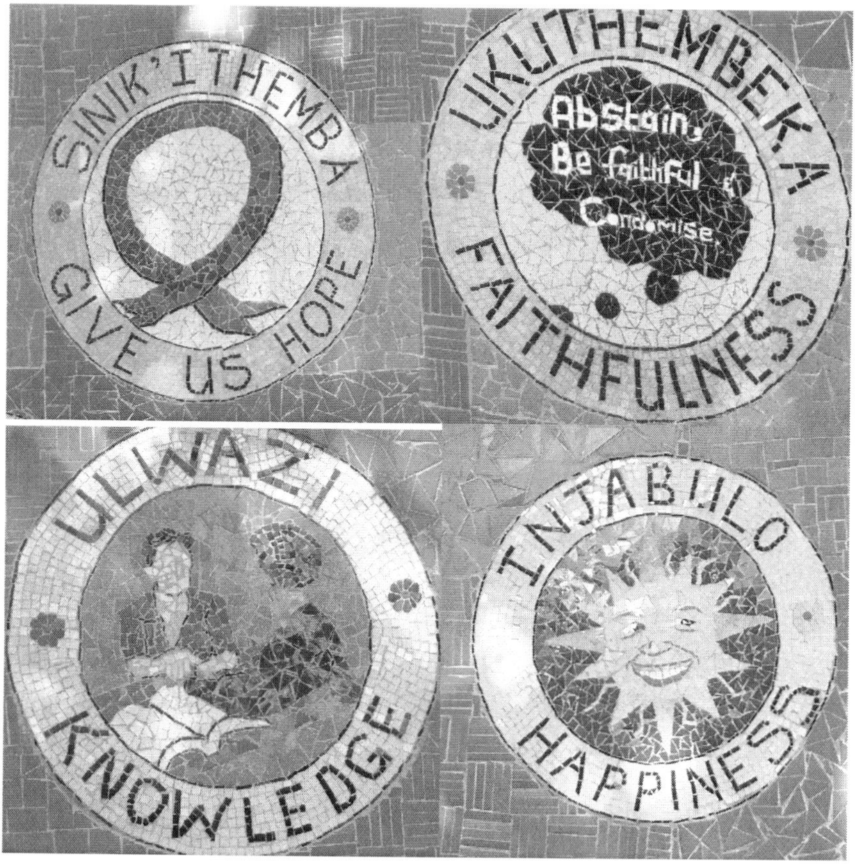

Figure 2.2 Mosaics made by the Sinikithemba Support Group members.

Other skills taught in the support group were woodworking and wood burning; even a computer literacy program was introduced. About half the proceeds from these projects went to the individuals who had produced specific objects, and about half was reserved to provide treatment for sick members.

WORKING AND SINGING: AN AFRICAN PHENOMENON THAT GAVE BIRTH TO A CHORAL ENSEMBLE

Much has been documented and written about the use of music to accompany work in African communities (Bebey 1975: 11; Nketia 1974: 28–29; Weman 1960: 80–82). Even early European explorers documented instances of extemporaneous music making during work. In 1800, for instance, Mungo

Park described the hospitality he received in present-day Senegambia coastal region from a wealthy African woman who engaged in the textile business and employed several young women to work at her enterprise to the accompaniment of songs.

> The rites of hospitality being thus performed toward a stranger in distress, my worthy benefactress, pointing to the mat, and telling me I might sleep there without apprehension, called to the female part of her family, who had stood gazing on me all the while in fixed astonishment, to resume their task of spinning cotton, in which they continued to employ themselves [a] great part of the night. They lightened their labor by songs, one of which was composed extempore, for I was myself the subject of it. It was sung by one of the young women, the rest joining in a sort of chorus: The air was sweet and plaintive, and the words literally translated, were these. "The winds roared, and the rains fell:—The poor white man, faint and weary, came and sat under the tree: He has no mother to bring him milk; no wife to grind his corn. *Chorus.* Let us pity the white man; no mother has he, &c. &c.[3]

Steve Biko observed in 1971 how European tourists in South Africa "watch with amazement the synchrony of music and action as African[*s*] working at a road side use their picks and shovels with well-timed precision to the accompaniment of a background song" (2004: 46). Central to Africans' use of music to accompany work is more than just the need to lighten the burden of work, or even to facilitate productivity, but "to share the burdens and pleasures of the work" as a communal experience (2004: 46).

Singing comprised an integral part of the activity of the Sinikithemba Support Group as its members worked on their projects. In an interview with Xolani Zulu, he described the process in these words.

> People were doing different things for income generations, like beadworks, craftwork, any handwork you can think of, in order to raise funds for their circumstances. So what happened, they started to sing when they are in groups, as mostly we Africans we used to do. When we are sad, we sing; when we are happy, we sing. Whenever we gather, we sing, you see.

It was in the context of the income-generating projects that the Siphithemba Choir was born. All choir members speak passionately about the times when they hummed hymn tunes and sang gospel songs while working at their projects. According to Phakamile Shabane, a female member of the choir, "We used to sing all the time, and everyone can sing any part they like. But it always sounded good." Another member Nomusa Mpanza testified about times when passersby on McCord Street would stop to listen to the sonorities of the group as its members worked at their tasks.

The environment of work performed to the accompaniment of song created yet another musical consciousness for members, but this time it was a consciousness that would permanently alter the dynamics of the group. According to Mrs. Mhlongo, "the group sang so well, and sometimes we even shed tears."

Asked why the tears, she explained that the songs they sang were sometimes emotional because they spoke to their individual experiences of being HIV-positive and being rejected by friends and families. She contemplated what to do to preserve the memory of a group that had functioned so much like a family. She feared that some of them would not survive long, and it would be worthwhile having something tangible to preserve their memory. According to her, at this time, she was already ruminating on turning the group into a choir, and she in fact expressed the desire to make a CD recording of the group's favorite tunes.

Their singing was not always melancholic. Nomusa and Phakamile attest to instances when their songs were upbeat, especially when they sang Zulu folksongs and gospel tunes that speak of courage in the face of adversity. Nomusa said the day that changed everything was sometime in early 1998, when the group had finished its work for the day and spent several more hours singing and dancing. "It was like we all went crazy that day, and everybody was watching us. So Nonhlanhla [Mrs. Mhlongo] suggested maybe we should form a choir." Thus, at Mrs. Mhlongo's suggestion, the support group formally became a choir, and it soon began performing at events in the hospital. The formation of the choir transformed the support group into a tri-functional entity—an HIV/AIDS support group, a microeconomic project, and a choral ensemble, all under the name Sinikithemba.

THE CHOIR AND THE AIDS CLINIC

McCord Hospital served as a testing site for a CD4/Viral Load research project, sponsored by the Center for AIDS Research at the Massachusetts General Hospital and Harvard Medical School, under the leadership of professor Bruce Walker. Many of the Sinikithemba Support Group members were participants in the project. By 1998, the success of the HIV/AIDS project at the hospital was drawing international attention, and there was a decision to erect a special AIDS clinic there. Sheila Davis, director of the Global Nurse Training Program at Harvard Medical School, who was helping to coordinate the building of the clinic, spoke to Mrs. Mhlongo about raising funds to help build the clinic. By then, the choir had already been formed, and so the group was deployed to help raise funds for the clinic by performing at major events at the hospital and around Durban.

The group had no trained conductor at the time, and accordingly its voices were not "polished," as Mrs. Mhlongo and Phumlani, the choir director, described them. Hence, Mrs. Mhlongo brought Phumlani Kunene to train and to conduct the choir. Phumlani had been a member of the support group, but had not frequently attended its meetings because of his employment. He was a trained teacher and a graduate of Westville College, now a campus of the University of KwaZulu-Natal, and had experience in conducting grade-school choirs. Upon arriving at the choir, he observed that the group had only one male voice. To balance the voice parts, he approached and brought on board two of his childhood friends, Xolani Zulu and Sizwe Ndlela. The three had been together as friends and musicians since their secondary-school days. As teenagers, they had performed in gospel choirs together and had sung in Afro-jazz vocal groups. They had produced their own records, and in some instances had worked with other recording artists. Sizwe was skilled on the keyboard and in dance choreography, while Xolani was noted for his strong bass voice and creative performance style; he played the electric bass and drum sets. These three worked together in developing the Siphithemba Choir.

Through local and international tours, the choir helped the hospital raise enough funds to complete the building of the AIDS clinic. The clinic is named Sinikithemba AIDS Clinic after the support group and the choir, and it stands as testimony to the success of the initiative to start the support group and transform it into a choral ensemble.

CHOIR OVERSEAS TOURS AND CONTINUED GROWTH

In 2002, executives of Church World Service—the international mission wing of the American Congregational Church, and the same body that had founded the Adams Mission in Amanzintonti in 1884 and the McCord Hospital in 1909—visited Durban with the plan of entering into a partnership program with McCord Hospital on HIV/AIDS. During the visit, they were thrilled at the resilience and exuberance shown by the choir members in their musical performance. They pledged to send Tim Janis, a White gospel artist, pianist, and composer from the state of Maine to work with the group. In the same year, he visited Durban, gave a benefit concert with the choir at the Durban City Hall, and recorded the album *A Thousand Summers* with the group, together with another group called Imilonji KaNtu. The proceeds from the sale of the CD recording were donated toward the funding of "African-run HIV/AIDS treatment and education projects" (Janis 2002). In December of 2002, sponsored by the Church World Service, the choir traveled to the United States, where it performed in churches and schools in the New York and Boston areas, raising awareness about HIV/AIDS and raising funds to provide antiretroviral treatments for support-group members. During this trip, professor Bruce Walker, who heads the Center for AIDS Research at Massachusetts General Hospital, observed the enthusiasm with which the choir's performances were being received in Massachusetts. He ensured that the choir would return to the United States in February of 2003 for the Tenth Conference on Retroviruses and Opportunistic Infections in Boston. Following that, the choir toured the United States regularly, visiting schools and churches in the cities of New York, Boston, Philadelphia, Washington, Hollywood in California, Chicago, and Indianapolis. During these trips, they have been presented with significant and symbolic gifts, including a replica of the liberty bell in Philadelphia, in recognition of their contribution to humanity in the fight against HIV/AIDS. In California, the Mayor of Hollywood presented the choir with the key to the city. Also, the choir has toured the United Kingdom with Sir Elton John, a renowned popular-music performer.

Back home in South Africa, the choir continued to raise its voice in educating and mobilizing communities against the disease by singing in hospital, community, and church social-action events and campaigns for AIDS education and treatment. It has several CD recordings to its name, including *A Thousand Summers* with Tim Janis *Sinikithemba Choir: Living Hope.* Two film documentaries have been made on the choir, including *Ithemba-Hope,* by Keefe Murren and Nelson Walker (2004); and *Raising their Voices: The Sinikithemba Choir,* by Shawn Hainsworth (2005).

In early 2006, the management of McCord Hospital determined that the choir had become large and strong enough to function independently; therefore, the choir separated from the hospital and renamed itself Siphithemba (We Give Hope or We Have Hope). The new name is slightly different from the original one, but it continues to echo the message of hope.

Although the group had separated from the hospital by the time I began working with them, they remain an important element in the McCord Hospital's HIV and AIDS work. Some members of the choir were still employed at the hospital's as HIV/AIDS counselors during the course of this research, and many continue to receive treatment at the hospital at a subsidized rate, while they also continue to participate in the ongoing AIDS-related research that uses McCord as a research site. They still get invited to perform at hospital events thereby maintaining close relationship with the hospital. Ultimately the Siphithemba Choir's story is intertwined with the story of McCord hospital and would not have been possible outside of such a space where human health is construed as intricately connected with human spirituality and the salvation of the human soul.

NOTES

1. Institute for International Medicine (INMED), "McCord Hospital, Durban, South Africa," www.inmed.us/training_sites/mccord_hospital_south_africa.asp.

2. Neither Mrs. Mhlongo nor any support-group member could tell with certainty the exact date of the first support-group meeting, but there is consensus that it was in late 1997, barely one year after Mrs. Mhlongo's arrival at McCord.

3. Reproduced in Southern 1983: 5–6.

Chapter 3

Music and Epidemics in South Africa[1]

The rhetoric of "the next struggle" that was introduced by late Nelson Mandela into the language of public discourse on HIV/AIDS in South Africa allowed students of music of AIDS and health in general to foreground current studies with analyses of the fallouts of the apartheid politics and how that impacted the current experience of the AIDS epidemic. This is particularly evident in what I discussed as the creative and expressive responses to the HIV/AIDS situation in chapter 1. I also suggested as will be shown throughout this work) that the apartheid story remains a history that looms large in the experience of HIV/AIDS in South Africa against which the music of the Siphithemba Choir must be appreciated especially when issues such as the politics of culture, race, and Black identity are addressed in their music. Yet, Zulu and Black South African social and political struggle extends beyond the sphere of secular politics into the sphere of public health.

In the course of this research, I tried to examine the history of disease epidemics in South Africa and to see if there are precedents of musical responses to public health situations that maybe juxtaposed with the current HIV/AIDS experience. In the process, I uncovered musical examples in previous epidemics, which parallel certain examples of current musical articulations of people's experience of HIV/AIDS, especially the music of the Siphithemba Choir.

In this chapter, I provide a historiography of music in times of epidemics stretching over a period of 300 years. Over this period, the territory we know today as the Republic of South Africa experienced several epidemics, including Smallpox (1713 to early 1900s); Rinderpest Epizootic (1896–1903); Malaria epidemic (1904); Influenza (1918 to late 1920s); and of course the HIV/AIDS (1982 to present). Cultural ways of responding to these epidemics could be gleaned.[2] I focus however on smallpox and influenza, especially because it is in these two that I have found extant responses of musical significance so far. These include a nineteenth-century folkloric sketch that contained references to music in the context of the smallpox epidemic, and a major musical composition by Reuben Caluza, a renowned South African composer and music educator written in response to the influenza epidemic. Despite the rarity of musical examples, analyses of the song examples placed against the background of the sociocultural contexts in which they were performed and or composed tell a lot about the people and their experiences of the diseases that affected their communities. I wish to juxtapose these with another contemporary choral work on HIV/AIDS by Lihle Biata in order to begin to reveal parallel articulations of disease experience, which will also ultimately illuminate some of the issues that I will be addressing about the music of the Siphithemba Choir going forward.

By juxtaposing case studies of musical responses to historical smallpox and influenza epidemics with the current use of music in the HIV/AIDS experience, I explore the meanings that people make of their experiences of diseases. I suggest that Siphithemba's music share commonalities with the songs that were created in previous epidemics in regard to the sociocultural constructions of meanings around disease epidemics. This is seen especially in articulations of the loss of traditional values, commentaries on faith and religion, and the performance of ethnic and racial identities. By positing a close reading of the song examples, I suggest that socio-cultural factors such as race and ethnicity, economics and spirituality comprise important frameworks for constructing meanings around the issue of health and in the context of epidemics.

Once again, my use of historiography in this chapter follows in the footsteps of earlier ethnomusicologists who have suggested that research on music could play a role in reconstructing history (Merriam 1967), thus permitting comparisons and interpretations that reveal larger ideas or trends shaping present events (Danielson 1997). In her study of the sacred music of South African indigenous churches, Carol Muller suggested that certain kinds of music could constitute archival practices, since their stylistic features contain repositories of history in both literate and pre-literate contexts (2002: 410). Relying on Jacques Derrida's reading on the Freudian notion of the psychic economy as a relationship between memory and archive, Muller argued, for example, that Isaiah Shembe's musical compositions and recommended performance practice constituted "retention of [African] cultural identity as a form of resistance to colonization" (2002: 426). When re-examined in present-day circumstances, the songs amount to historicizing gestures that illuminate the cultural meanings embedded in contemporary performances, and underscore the social dynamics that pervade present-day post-apartheid South Africa's political and religious climate.

In the light of the above, therefore, a close reading of musical responses to epidemics reveals something of music's artistic commitment to archeological inquiry (Mercer 1990: 7–9), in this case the archeology of health. Emergent scholarship on music and epidemics has proven informative in this regard. Relying on the blues song collections by John Morgan, a professor at the City University of New York Medical School, Dan Baum reconstructed the history and impact of the "Jake Leg" (denatured alcohol-based paralysis) outbreak in the United States in the early 1930s. He argued that but for a number of Black Southern Blues singers who encoded their and their communities' experiences of the condition in song, "the [jake leg] epidemic would have probably remained forgotten" (2003: 8). Similarly, Linda and Michael Hutcheon (1996) examined the repeated representations of plagues in nineteenth-and twentieth-century operas. According to the Hutcheons, the representations reveal complex and dynamic interactions between medical and cultural meanings. Such dynamic interactions produce metaphors, which they suggest must be "historicized" by placing them in the context of their past use (1996: 197). The authors thus argue that the metaphors bring fresh insight to the social constructions and cultural meanings being assigned to the current global AIDS pandemic, and will perhaps afford insight in future epidemics.

The historiographical research at the center of this chapter reveals parallels between South African outbreaks of smallpox (1713–1900), influenza (1918–1920), and HIV/AIDS (1982 to present) in three major areas. First, songs from all three epidemics address the loss of traditional values, including loss of the sense of community and moral rectitude. Second, the songs hint at prevailing sociocultural and political dynamics (the interracial acrimony between Whites and Blacks) that shaped the conversations around community health. And finally, each epidemic includes songs that capture issues of witchcraft and stigma. The parallel manifestations thus help to answer questions such as whether we can see any meaningful continuities addressing how people deal with diseases over time, especially those of epidemiological magnitude, and whether those continuities could explain the ways in which Black South Africans are responding to HIV and AIDS. With regard to the Siphithemba Choir specifically, I suggest first, that their music, like those produced in previous epidemics, comprise the expressions of individual members' experiences as microcosmic reflection of that of their community. Together they reveal consistencies in historically and culturally informed perceptions and interpretations of disease in South Africa, which in turn shape the nature of local responses to the disease. Second, examining the musical articulation of the people's experiences of diseases reveals how, by virtue of its history, South Africa's public health is entangled with the nation's politics—thus underscoring a set of consistent sociocultural dynamics that characterize health discourses in each historical period.

SMALLPOX

Smallpox hit the geographical territory of what is known today as South Africa at several intervals between the early 1700s and the close of the nineteenth century. According to a nineteenth-century historical account, smallpox first appeared in the Cape Colony in March 1713 when a handful of African women in a slave lodge in the Cape were forced to handle laundry materials of previously sick crewmen of a Dutch East India Company vessel on passage from India. As a consequence, the disease entered the African population, and by May and June of that same year, "there was hardly a family in the town that had not someone sick or dead. Among the free Blacks the mortality was very great, the Hottentots suffering most. Whole kraals [walled villages] disappeared without leaving a single representative" (*British Medical Journal*, henceforth BMJ 1900: 595).

A second, more severe smallpox outbreak hit South Africa in the winter of 1755, "introduced by a homeward bound fleet from Ceylon" (BMJ 1900: 596). Although Edward Jenner had discovered the smallpox vaccine by 1796, it did not receive regular distribution in South Africa until about the 1890s.[3] Thus, outbreaks continued to plague the region well into the late 1800s, causing drastic demographic depression in African communities. Unfortunately, no detailed records were kept on the impact of the disease in the African communities except accounts written by volunteer medical practitioners and missionaries.[4] It appears from these accounts that the virus wreaked its worst havoc in African communities between the 1850s and the 1880s. In response to direct communication from Surgeon Major Pringle in 1884, Havelock Sturge, the district surgeon for Xalanga in the Cape Colony, provided a gloomy picture of the smallpox epidemic and its impact:

> The mortality was greater, perhaps, than it would otherwise have been, owing to the insufficient care the people had. The lot of the unfortunates shut in the quarantine was pitiable in the extreme. In one instance, out of more than thirty enclosed every male died; and the girls, while themselves stricken, had to dig the graves and bury their relations. (BMJ 1889: 353)

Two Basotho song performances addressing smallpox during this time survive, as translated by the French missionary and explorer Thomas Arbousset (1810–1887) who worked in Southern Africa between 1832 and 1860.[5] The Scottish poet and folklorist John Crombie later published the texts of the songs in an 1890 collection of poetic and folkloric sketches.[6] The songs speak volumes about the way the people interpreted as well as imagined the impact of the disease in their communities.

We are left outside,
We are left for sorrow,
We are left to despair,
Which increases our misery!
Oh, that there were a refuge in heaven!
That there were a pot there and a fire!
That there were found a place for me!
Oh, that I had wings to fly thither!

A second song text reads:

I feel pity when I see smallpox making its ravages and spoiling the face.
Here at home in the village we no longer live.
We no longer are kind to each other, even among relatives.
It is the fault of this terrible disease.
This disease is truly terrible, my Lord!
It has driven the son-in-law from his home;
He goes, but returns with cruel words.
The old woman comes this way. . . .
She is turned out; she goes away and dies in the bush.

We may never know what these songs sounded like, but Crombie's description of Arbousset's account provides some degree of insight to the performance practice. The first song is a wailing song that was performed by women. In the second song performed by men, according to Arbousset, "old men limp about, simulating pain" depicting the physical bodily impact of smallpox.

Even without actual sonic documentation, the texts of the two songs have much to say about the social impact of the disease, especially regarding the loss of traditional values. First, the two songs suggest the existence of a stigmatizing attitude meted out against women who may have been infected by the disease. The texts indicate that those suffering from the disease were stigmatized in a manner akin to witchcraft accusation (see Berglund 1989) in which the accused could be ostracized, procedurally removed from the homestead, and sometimes even beaten to death.[7] It is not clear why women are the victims of the social attitudes evident in the two songs, but it is certainly consistent with the ways in which many societies typically associate women with witchcraft activities (Roach 2013; Chadhuri 2012: 1213–1234).[8] The second song represents smallpox in anthropomorphic terms. In lines two through six, smallpox is described not just as an agent of destruction for the body, but also for the people's sense of community and mutual interdependency.

Here at home in the village we no longer live.
We no longer are kind to each other, even among relatives.
It is the fault of this terrible disease.

Is the personification of the epidemic in the song a literary practice with mere surface structure meaning, or does it also index a particular social dynamic? In exploring this question, I wish to point out two important issues of sociocultural relevance about the epidemics at this time. First, Africans widely distrusted Europeans as honest interveners in the plague. Traditional healers and diviners (Izinyanga and Izangoma respectively) postulated that Europeans could not provide an effective remedy to the spread of the disease. Hence, they counseled members of their communities against vaccinations even when Africans trained in Western medicine served as providers, for they were perceived as co-conspirators in the plague's transmission. They instead encouraged their patients to "swallow a pint or two of stewed roots as a charm against the disease . . ." (Sturge 1889: 353). This act of distrust accounted for the difficulties and setbacks in the vaccination initiatives in the Xalanga district of the Transkei (Sturge in the 1889 BMJ).

A second, related issue, is that Europeans gradually reached the point of associating the smallpox with Black bodies, thus prompting the call to tighten South African segregationist policies as a means of protecting Europeans. A September 3, 1887 report in the British Medical Journal reads:

> It is reported that small-pox has attacked the natives in the Matatiele district, and that in some of the locations all the huts have persons suffering badly. . . . It is a curious and happy circumstance that no person of European extraction appears to have been afflicted with it. The operation of the Pass Law [allowing Black South Africans to travel within the country] is to be suspended for a time, with the hope of limiting the spread of the disease. (BMJ 1887: 521)

These clear mutual distrust between Africans and Europeans regarding who was spreading the disease offers a gloss on the aforementioned song text: articulating Africans' experience of smallpox as an agent of divisiveness, the cause of the loss of traditional values, and a harbinger of social disintegration. The disease, so personified, also parallels the perception of the European as a divider and conqueror, affording the virus the ability to cause destruction by disrupting the sense of family and community. Both Europeans and smallpox, in this view, deprive the African population of its agency and ability to maintain their sense of community and social cohesion.

THE 1918 INFLUENZA

The first quarter of the twentieth century once again marked an era of great pestilence in South Africa, especially the influenza of 1918–1920. Part of the pandemic that killed between twenty and forty million people worldwide, Influenza entered Southern Africa in a way that recalled the smallpox epidemics: ships of infected European soldiers returning from the First World War landed at the major ports of Durban and Cape Town; and from there the disease spread rapidly around the urban centers and into the rural areas (see Ranger 1988; Phillips 1990). As with the smallpox epidemic, we have only general records of the rate and impact of the epidemic in the Black South African population, thanks mainly to the government's indifference to the health status of those who lived in urban slums and the rural areas (see Parnell 1991: 271–288). What is more significant is how Africans themselves responded to the epidemic, especially in the domains of spirituality and artistic expression. The case of Reuben Tholakele Caluza (1895–1969) acclaimed as South Africa's foremost composer of his generation (Erlmann 1995), presents a particularly illustrative example.

Born into a musically inclined Christian family, Reuben attended and later taught at the Zulu Ohlange Christian Institute, where his musical prowess was boosted under John L. Dube's tutelage (see Coplan 1985: 70–71; Erlmann 1991: 118–119). Famous for his nationalistic compositions, Caluza's large collection of songs written in tonic sol-fa and published by the Lovedale Institution Press were used to instill a sense of direction in his Natal and South African urban Black audiences, and they often addressed the social, political, and economic experiences of the people. Around 1919, with South Africa still under the scourge of the influenza, Caluza composed a song titled "Influenza 1918," which the Lovedale Institution Press published as part of the sol-fa leaflet series.[9] The song included in his 1930 recording project with his Double Quartet at the HMV studio in London, with Caluza himself on the piano and as director. The recording was remastered by Paul Vernon and Charlie Crump and rereleased in a compact disc in 1992 by The Heritage Music label. Contained in the recording along with "influenza" are other songs by Caluza and his arrangements of pre-existing folk songs, which "present a vivid portrait of one of the most turbulent phases in black South African history" (see Erlmann 1995, CD liner note). These include "Umteto we Land Act" which is the recorded version of his "Si Lu Sapo or iLand Act" (to be commented on later) and "Sanibona" which also makes partial reference to the influenza epidemic. The compositional style of "influenza" shows clear Western influence: English hymn-style four-part harmony, verse-chorus format, and the use of periodic chromaticism especially in the refrain sections.

"INFLUENZA"[10]

A

Ngonyaka ka nineteen eighteen
Saqedwa ukufa esikubiza ngokuti kuyi influenza

Yazi qeda izihlobo esizitandayo
Omama na obaba no Sisi no Bhuti
Kwemnyimizi kwaqotula a kwasala' muntu
Kwatat'intombi nensizwa,
Kwaziketel'ezinhle
Kwatata na mabhungu ayebukeka kahle
Kwatata majongosi
Kwatata namatshitshi,
Kwatat'izingoduso ezazetenjisiwe
Kwatat'omakotshana,
Kanye nabakwenyama
Kwangati kuku n'if'elimnyama
Pezu kwalomhlaba

B

Kwas'ongati izolanda intombi nensizwa
Yaba ngcono kwabadala yabeqed'abasha
Omame na obaba bashi y'intandane zihlupeka
Zinosizi zingancedwa 'muntu.
Noko namhla sesikohlwa usiz'olukulu,
Kwakunjenake endulo
Kwababey'eKanana
Kwati nxabehlupeka,
Baqal'ukuzisola.
Kwakutinxa bebusa behamba ngentokozo
Bangacabangi luto ngay'ong' umenzi wabo.
Kwapumelela labo ababekonza yena.
Iningi labanye lafa lapela kona l'ehlane,
Siya niyala nsizwa
Siya niyala ntombi
Musa n'ukuvumel'inhliziyo
Ngoba ayigcweli.

A

In the year 1918
We're killed by the disease called influenza
Which finished our beloved relatives
Mothers, fathers, sisters and brothers
In other households no one was left
It took young women and men
It chose the beautiful ones
It even took the good looking men
It took the teenagers
It took even the young maidens
It took the engaged ladies

It took the strummers (bridesmaids)
Even the grooms
It was like there was a black cloud
Over the earth

B

Just as it comes to collect young women and men
It burned out the elders, while it finished the youth
Mothers, fathers left the orphans
Miserable with no one to help
So today we've forgotten the great help
It was like this long ago
With those who went to Canaan
When they faced difficulties
They felt sorry for their wrong doings [They regret]
When things go well they go with joy
They didn't think about their creator
Only they were successful who worshiped him
Many others died in the wilderness
We warn you men
We warn you young women
Do not follow your heart
Because of non-satisfaction [lust]

"Influenza 1918" could be analyzed as musical binary form in A/A^1. The musical sections do not necessarily correspond to the text, as the textual placing overlap in the musical sections. The Text of the A section paints a picture of the impact of the epidemic in the African population, the message of which carries into lines sixteen through nineteen in the A^1 section. While Caluza's chronicling mirrors the documentation by other scholars regarding the global onslaught of the disease among people in their prime (between ages 20 and 40, see Crosby 1976: 215; Nicholson et al. 1998: 11; Johnson and Mueller 2002: 106; Langford 2002: 2), he differs from them in his observation that the epidemic also decimated the elderly population, thus differentiating the African communities' experience from that of other global contexts.

It is in the A^1 section that Caluza made the most significant poetic statement. He employed the biblical hermeneutical strategy of typology analysis, in which the events of Israelite history are interpreted as prefiguring modern events. In Caluza's lyricism, the influenza epidemic was likened to the punishment in the biblical exodus event, which God visited upon the Hebrews for abandoning His covenant with them (Ex. 32: 35; Num. 14: 26–38). Hence Caluza called for repentance and change in behavior using the medium of his song.

Contemporary sources affirm that Caluza's interpretation reflects a common attitude about the disease, at least among Zulu and other Nguni Christians. The message in the song parallels that of Nontetha Nkwenkwe, a Xhosa prophetess and influential millenarian preacher who in the 1920s interpreted the epidemic as God's punishment for the growing immorality and mischief among Africans who thoughtlessly embraced Western and colonial lifestyles (Edgar and Sapire 2000: 8). Nkwenkwe warned that only penitence would prevent a total obliteration of the population of her people in the Ciskei and Transkei, and all over South Africa. It is not clear whether Caluza intended this song to be interpreted or even performed as religious music or within a religious space. Nonetheless, the sermonic nature of the song, especially in the A^1 section, and the overall English hymn-like nature of the song speaks to his Presbyterian upbringing. One might argue that the correlation between the hymn-like compositional style of the song and its sermonic lyricism is intentional, especially because anthems are known to be historically composed in the English church with a homiletic functional role. Nontetha Nkwenkwe's interpretation of the thoughtless embrace of Western and colonial lifestyles also saw parallels in other published songs by Caluza, namely "Sannibona" (We Greet You) and "Intandane" (Orphan) that were composed in about 1920. These songs were addressed particularly to South Africa's urban Black population, who Caluza believed had become disconnected from their rural roots, resulting in their loss of the sense of traditional values and uncritical embrace of the frivolous Western lifestyles. The African value of commitment to family and community, as he saw it, was threatened, most significantly during moments of great anguish such as those unleashed by the influenza epidemic.

On another level, disputes over land ownership and eminent domain may have also shaped how Africans responded to the influenza epidemic. The outbreak came barely five years after the 1913 Land Act, which laid the blueprint for governmental appropriation of seventy percent of the territory for a small White population; Reuben Caluza responded with a song titled "Si Lu Sapo or iLand Act."[11] Similar to the responses to the smallpox epidemic, South African Blacks distrusted the Europeans and the White government's sincerity as interveners in the epidemic. Traditional healers and itinerant preachers dissuaded people from participating in government-sponsored inoculations, warning that the influenza was "a device of the Europeans to finish off the Native races of South Africa" (Christian Express 1918: 85). Reuben Caluza's song, which called on all Africans to unite in defense of their land, could have contributed to, or at least coordinated with, Africans' understanding of land as an important factor in public discourses about the influenza epidemic. His songs thus reflected the ways in which Africans thought about the spiritual and material causes of disease, providing insight into the ways Africans responded on the ground.

THE HIV/AIDS: NEW EPIDEMIC, OLD ISSUES

In response to this new HIV/AIDS epidemic, individuals and groups have tended to reach back into the cultural resources that spurred them during the antiapartheid struggles as tools for combating the disease. I wish to show here some of the sociocultural dynamics and politics that find expression in music, revealing the lens through which Black South Africans view and interpret HIV and AIDS. I note once again as already cited in chapter 1 that there are several documentations on individual and musical groups that have been deploying music in the context of the current HIV/AIDS epidemic. I have also noted the scope of issues that are addressed in the musical examples, where majority tend to be focused on the use of music especially popular music as a form of grassroots education and mobilization. I draw from my own field research, which happened to be primarily choral music. While I worked primarily with the Siphithemba Choir, I had the opportunity to also document other song examples in churches and at choral-music festivals and competitions. It was through this means that I came to know about Lihle Biata and his compositions, some of which have been performed in KwaZulu-Natal and in the Eastern Cape.

Lihle Biata hails from Lusikisiki in the Mbizana district of the Eastern Cape. I heard Biata's song first in 2005 during a district level choral festival and competition at the Orient Theatre in East London where his song "Indiza Mtshini" (Flying Machine) was featured as a set piece for male voices. By the time I met with him at his Lusikisiki home in 2007, Biata had lost a whole collection of the AIDS songs that were meant to be an opus with up to fifteen movements on AIDS. I worked with him to salvage some of the songs by reassembling bits and pieces of his sol-fa manuscripts and by reaching out to some choirmasters who had performed one or two of his songs. By this means I was able to assess and analyze aspect of his songs some of which reveal striking similarities in thought pattern with songs in the previous epidemics. Two songs from the opus, "Inyala" (Indecency) and "Ilolo" (Wailing), especially illustrate the issues of the loss of traditional values and spirituality similar to the ones that were seen in music of smallpox and comparable to Reuben Caluza's influenza song.

'Inyala' Indecency
Yini le, idunga ibulale?
Yini le, ixhaphaxhapha isizwe?
Kwanele, kwanele yini?
Satshabalala okwe zilwanyana
Nali-nya-la lothando.
Sizi Nkedama O'thixo

Sashi ywa ngaBazali
Ngeli' inyala.
Yayi ntl' indalo izintombi zazihlowa
Sakhala iSalukazi Nal' inyala
S'yapheli Sizwe- nguwe
Tha bakho, kwanele.

Sermonette

Abantu bakuthi bafa okweMpukani ngenxa yoThando
Sakhala isalukazi sathi Linyala eli.
What is this, that defiles and kills?
What is this, that tears away the nation?
It's enough, it's enough why?
We die like animals
Here is indecency called love.
We are Orphans, Oh, God
We have been left by parents
Through this indecency
There was beauty of nature [when] girls were inspected
The old woman cries here is indecency
The Nation is devastated- by you
As you take them, enough.

Sermonette

Our people die like Flies because of Love
The Old woman cries and says, this is indecency

Ilolo Text, *By Lihle Biata*

Measures 1–7, all voice parts sing the same texts

Bahleli ngasekunene
Bahleli bejabulile
Ba ngishi ya ngi lele abazili bam

Measures 8–12 different voice parts are assigned different texts as shown

Sop/Alt. Siyathakathana, siyamonclana
Uphin' umama, uphin tata?
Sukhalamntwana wam
Ten/Bas. Kwane le! Kwane le!)
All. Yosi gubakuzekuthini?

Measures 13–16 different voice parts are assigned different texts as shown

Sop Yinina!senzeni-kuMdali
Yinina!senzeni-kuThixo
Alto Ziphin'izimbongi-zibhodle
Aphin'Amagqirha-ajoje
Ten. Hoyi Nina!
Hoyi Nina
Sukhalamntwanawam
Bas. Unga shonangalekukhalinyembezi
Unga shonangale-kukhal'izijwili
Baph'inabazali bami
All. Yozi gubakuzekuthini?

Measures 17–19, Ten.1/Ten.2/Bas.

Thethele la Thixo mkhulu
Usathana uyazenzela

Measures 20–29, different voice parts are assigned different texts as shown

Sop/Alt. Sicela sicela bobakho
Ten/Bas. Amandla ngawakho
Nobungcwa lisabezulu bobakho

Measures 30–63, textual uniformity in all voice parts

Kwa kuhle kha ya sidlilisa
Sakhal'iSalukazi yantlingane
Lak'shoni la ngandoshonaphi mina
Ih, ih, xakunjenanje
Siya ya eNyamazana
Sizi nkedama O'thixo
Sashiywa ngabazali ngisemncane
Dala imithetho yakho kulomhlaba Thixo

They are seated at the right hand (of God)
They are seated happily
My parents left me sleeping

Measures 8–12 different voice parts are assigned different texts as shown

Sop/Alt. We bewitch and are jealous of one another
Where is mother, where is father

Don't cry my baby
Ten/Bas. Enough! Enough!
All. How long shall this be?

Measures 13–16 different voice parts are assigned different texts as shown

Sop What have we done to God?
What have we done to the Lord?
Alto Where are the poets?
Where are the wise?
Ten. Oh You!
Oh You!
Don't cry my child
Bas. You go there, there are tears
You go there, there is [sorrowful] weeping
Where are my parents?

All. How long shall this be?

Measures 17–19, Ten.1/Ten.2/Bas.

Forgive Almighty God
It is the devil's doing

Measures 20–29, different voice parts are assigned different texts as shown

Sop/Alt. We pray, we beg you
Ten/Bas. All power is yours
And to you belongs the heavenly holiness

Measures 30–63, textual uniformity in all voice parts

Its better to play in the homestead
The grandmother cries out to the children
When the sun sets, whence do I go?
When it is like this
We go to Nyamazana
We're orphans oh Lord
We ought to be by our parents when I'm young
Your law Lord is old in this world

The two songs are both through-composed, and Biata indicates that they be performed moderately slow *"con lacrimosa."* They differ slightly, however, in harmonic texture and performance. Inyala is homophonic and can be repeated with humming, over which a solo voice can improvise with a

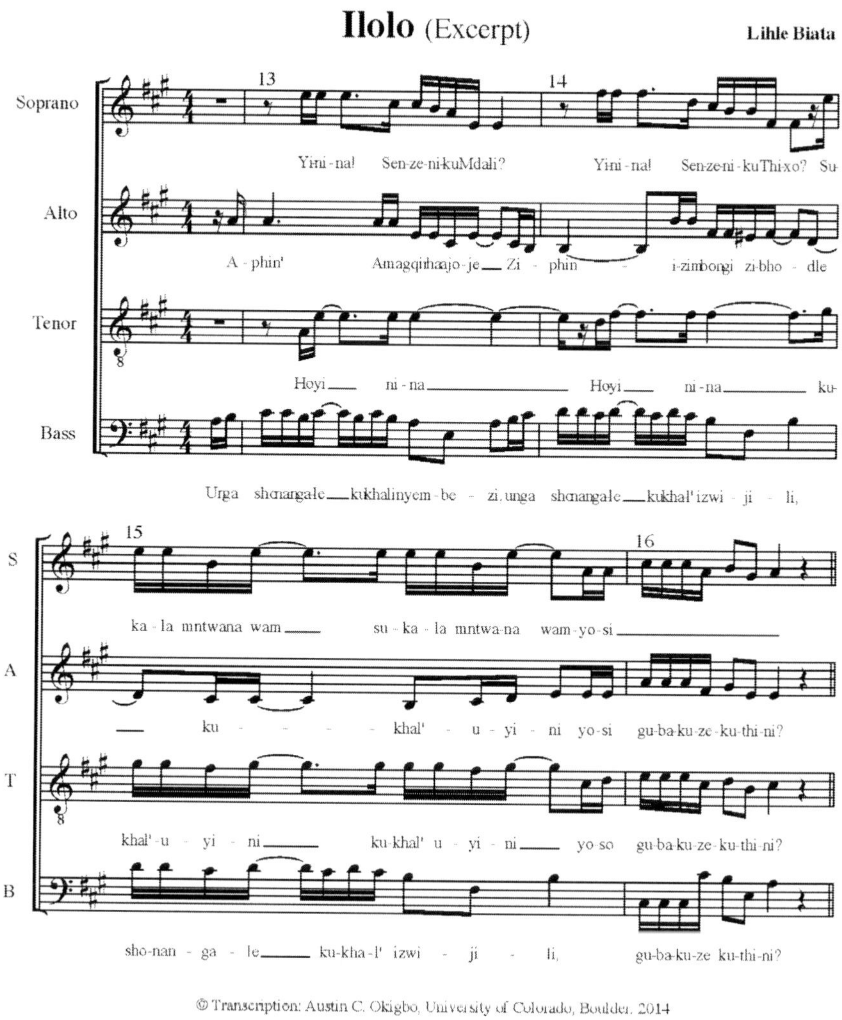
Ilolo (Excerpt)
Lihle Biata
Soprano
Alto
Tenor
Bass
13
14
Yini - na! Sen-ze-ni-kuMdali? Yini - na! Sen-ze-ni - kuThi-xo? Su-
A - phin' Amagqirhaajo - je Zi - phin i-zimbongi zi-bho - dle
Hoyi ni - na Hoyi ni - na ku-
Unga shonangale kukhalinyem - be - zi, unga shonangale kukhal' izwi - ji - li,
15
16
S
A
T
B
ka - la mntwana wam su - ka - la mntwa-na wam - yo - si
ku - khal' - u - yi - ni yo-si gu-ba-ku-ze-ku-thi-ni?
khal' - u - yi - ni ku-khal' u - yi - ni yo-so gu-ba-ku-ze-ku-thi-ni?
sho-nan - ga - le ku-kha - l' izwi - ji - li, gu-ba-ku-ze ku-thi-ni?
© Transcription: Austin C. Okigbo, University of Colorado, Boulder. 2014

Figure 3.1 Excerpt of Lihle Biata's "Ilolo" showing polyphonic style.

sermonette[12] a la Black American gospel music delivery style. In contrast, Ilolo is polyphonic for the most part, whereby in some sections, Biata assigned different texts to different voice parts (see figure 3.1). The compositional technique applied in such sections as shown resulted in a seeming cacophony of voices representing people's expressions of different opinions and feelings about the AIDS problem. By so doing, Biata sonically captures the imagined sense of confusion and restlessness that AIDS brought into the lives of individuals, families, and the society at large.

In comparison to Reuben Caluza's "Influneza," Biata makes reference in both songs to the devastation and the decimation of the population caused by AIDS. While Siphithemba's songs as will be shown later framed the problem in racial/nationalistic terms, Biata followed a course similar to Reuben Caluza in lines 5 and 8 of Inyala by alleging divine causality due to indecent behavior. Immediately following that in lines 9 through 12, Biata pivots back to the traditional practice of virginity testing among the Nguni groups of South Africa, which was used to ensure that young girls did not engage in pre-marital sex. This part of the song echoes the message that will be heard in some of of Siphithemba's songs such as, "Isiyalo" and "Ikhalaphi." It is deducible from Biata's songs, that a loss of this traditional practice and value system is blamed at least partly for the onslaught of the AIDS pandemic. I have noted hereby that the current Zulu monarch, Nkosi Zwelithini, has argued for using the practice of virginity testing, which forms part of the *Umkhosi woMhlaba* (the annual royal reed dance festival) as a cultural tool for fighting the spread of HIV/AIDS. Also, as recent as January 2016, the Mayor of Uthukela in the KwaZulu-Natal Province, disclosed in an interview with the British Broadcasting Corporation (BBC), that her district has awarded scholarship to sixteen female university students which are conditional on them remaining virgins. The mayor Dudu Mazibuko defended her action amid criticisms by Rights groups that the aim is to "reduce HIV [and] AIDS and unwanted pregnancy" among young girls in the district. To retain the bursary however, the recipients, who have already received virginity tests as part of the annual Zulu reed ceremony, must provide proof of regular virginity tests.[13]

In line four of Ilolo, Biata introduced the issue of witchcraft and the mutual mistrust of one another in the community due to the epidemics in the soprano and alto parts, while the tenors and basses vigorously shouted *Enough!* The allusion here compares with the theme of social disintegration in the second song that was performed during the smallpox epidemic in the 1800s, so that HIV/AIDS, like smallpox, becomes once again an agent of divisiveness and community disintegration. Biata would not confirm whether he believes that HIV could be inflicted through the art of witchcraft. Instead, in a private conversation, he connected the social attitudes that have become attendant to the explosion of the AIDS pandemic—stigma and ostracism of HIV-positive members of the community by families and friends, as well as anger and hatred—as belonging to *ubuthakathi,* the witchcraft system. His suggestion that witchcraft causes members of a community to stone a person to death tacitly recalls the cold-blooded murder of Gugu Dlamini in 1998 in KwaMashu, outside of Durban, for publicly disclosing her HIV+ status on the Zulu radio station Radio Ukhozi. Some of the people who participated in her killing thought Gugu was a witch whose public disclosure of her

HIV+ status was simply witchcraft confession; she deserved, in their view, to be punished with ostracism and death—a punishment comparable to that which women suffered during the smallpox epidemic, as evidenced in the song examples.

Finally, in Ilolo, Biata devotes more space to asking how long God would punish the people, offering a prayer of repentance, and begging for forgiveness on behalf of the people. Why the prayer of repentance and plea for forgiveness? The myth that HIV/AIDS is a curse from God as punishment for the sins of people has been propagated by some evangelical preachers such as Billy Graham and Jerry Falwell (Kopelman 2002; Chikwem et al., 2003: 1). Similarly, there are several preachers in South Africa who allege divine causality in the spread of the HIV/AIDS, although it is arguable that none has gained notoriety like Nontetha Nkwenkwe who preached during the scourge of the 1918 influenza. Thus in South Africa some evangelical and Pentecostal churches refuse to introduce AIDS programs in their faith communities in the belief that morally responsible children of God cannot contract HIV. The situation wherefore HIV/AIDS is imagined as direct consequence of sin forms part of private and public conversations in the society, thus finding expression in Lihle Biata's songs.

SUMMARY AND CONCLUSION

My purpose in this chapter has been to juxtapose a close reading of songs in the current experience of HIV/AIDS in South Africa with musical responses in earlier epidemics. This historiographical approach helps to reveal the parallels in the songs, showing the sociocultural and political processes that shaped the health discourses under the various epidemics, thereby also revealing the persistence of social constructions in community experiences over time. In light of Carol Muller's discourse on songs as archives, we can appreciate the value of the musical productions under the onslaught of smallpox and influenza as repositories of memory and history, especially given the lack of other written documentation of community experiences during these epidemics. This study therefore participates in the discourse on music as memory and archive: first because the songs became the places of consignation of the memories of those who experienced the epidemics. The songs thus have the capacity to serve the purpose of remembering the past. Second, the songs participate in the value of the archive as casting historical light upon present circumstances. In this case, the parallels seen between the musical examples in the current experience of HIV/AIDS and previous epidemics—the sense of the loss of traditional values, spirituality, and interracial acrimony—become all the more evident. Third, in light of Derrida's postulation that the place of the archive "is a question of the future itself, a question of a response, . . . and of a responsibility for tomorrow" (1995: 36), this musical historiography provides a perspective that could be useful to understanding how responses to future epidemics continue persistent frameworks for constructing meanings around the issue of health.

Finally, the historiographical approach furthers the study of African music as communal action and experience, in which individuals who live a corporate life, or share common values and/or life experiences, use music making as a form of social intercourse, rendering a community ethos in performance (Nketia 1974: 21). In this vein, musical composition and performance as archival practice comprise narratives of communal history, and articulations of collective experience and memory. When individuals such as Reuben Caluza and Lihle Biata compose songs, they do so mainly as possessors of the power of artistic agency to articulate the collective experience of their communities. Through their works, we enter into their communities' matrix of meanings in the context of dire public health situations. In the light of the Hutcheons' suggestion that metaphors and representations present in music during various epidemics are "reminders of the power of disease in the larger social realms," (1996: 20), this chapter uncovers a musical angle to the folkloristics of health: especially that of the cycle of passing the blame, which often stem from stories, rumors, and conspiracy theories that are not based on reality. Folklorist/anthropologists Charles Briggs and public health scholar Clara Mantini-Briggs' study of the cholera epidemic in the delta region of Venezuela between 1992 and 1993 reveal how both racism and mutual distrust between the indigenous Warao and the mainstream population and public-policy officials who blamed the Warao for spreading the disease contributed to the devastation witnessed in the epidemic. The question they sought to answer in their study is why so many would die near the end of the twentieth century from an easily treatable bacterial infection associated with the premodern past. Drawing from evidence of their studies, the Briggses concluded, "[W]hen germs and race mix, however inadvertently, the result is often fatal" (2003: 5). Their findings compare with much of what I have found in this historical musical precedence in South Africa, which I tried to examine against the background of the sociocultural contexts in which the songs were produced. Most importantly and drawing from the evidence in the South African experience, I suggest that persistent sociocultural conditions produce similar results, namely how people interpret their experiences of disease epidemics and by extension how they respond to that experience. I therefore urge the reader to pay close attention and note the parallels in the culture and politics of health in the context of the South African HIV/AIDS experience and how these find expression in the music of the Siphithemba Choir.

NOTES

1. This chapter draws from a paper "South African Music in the History of Epidemics" being considered for publication in the Journal of Folklore Research in which I explored the issue of historicity and continuity in cultural meanings of health and disease, and in which I made the case for musical historiography as a means of reconstructing the sociocultural dimensions and folkloristics of health in the absence of written records of disease epidemics in human communities.

2. See for instance Benedict Carton, 2011 on the rinderpest plague that reached the southernmost tip of the continent in Natal and Zululand in 1896; also L'Abbe et al. on the typhoid epidemic that hit the mines of Kimberly and its environs.

3. Several Vaccination Acts were enacted in Britain, at least eight of them between 1840 and 1871. The enforcement of the Acts was however marred by the antivaccinationist movements that invoked conscientious objections championed by working-class liberalists against government interference in individual privacy, and reformists' theologically based revolt against "New Science" and scientific medicine (see Fenner et al. 1988: 270). The movements were replicated in some of the colonies including South Africa, so that the slow distribution of the vaccines became all the more compounded by Black South Africans' suspicion of the Europeans as dishonest interveners in the epidemics.

4. In a note on the epidemics of smallpox among Blacks of the Transkei contained in the February 16, 1889 issue of the British Medical Journal, Havelock Sturge, the former district surgeon, of Xalanga in the Cape Colony, revealed the routes, namely labor migrancy, by which the epidemics spread and wrecked its havoc in Black communities (BMJ 1889: 353). Most importantly he observed the lack of accurate records, suggesting therefore the difficulty in estimating "the number of people who suffered during the epidemic" (BMJ 353), such that "his numbers *which clearly reflected a bleak situation at the time* refer to those actually seen by [him]self" (BMJ 1889: 353).

5. Thomas Arbousset (1810–1887) was also noted for his interest in explorations, the reports of which earned him awards from the Geographical Society of Paris (see Spindler, Marc R. "Thomas Arbousset 1810 to 1887, Protestant Lesotho." *Dictionary of African Christian Biography* http://www.dacb.org/stories/lesotho/arbousset_thomas.html cited on 10/21/2012).

6. See Crombie, John W. 1890 [1891]. *Some Poets of the People in Foreign Lands*. London: Eliot Stock.

7. This social attitude is similar to, and partly accounted for the brutal public killing of Gugu Dlamini in 1998 in KwaMashu, outside of Durban for publicly disclosing her HIV+ status on the Zulu radio station Radio Ukhozi.

8. It also resembles the current gendered terms associated with sexually transmitted diseases in some African societies such as among the Shona in Zimbabwe and in Eastern Nigeria, which identify the female body as the bearer and transmitter of such diseases. In eastern Nigeria for example, radio broadcasters are known to use the expression *ọrịa nsi nwanyị*, which translates literally as "woman poison sickness."

9. See *Lovedale Sol-Fa Leaflets*, No. 11C, held at the Killie Campbell Africana Library, UKZN, Durban, South Africa.

10. Translated with the assistance of Phakamile Shabane.

11. See Lovedale sol-fa leaflets No. 1c by Lovedale Press, courtesy of the Killie Campbell Africana Library, UKZN, Durban, South Africa.

12. The term *sermonette* is used by Portia Maultsby to describe the ad lib vocal gestures that gospel artists use to establish rapport with their audience (Maultsby 2005: 329). I use the term to designate similar practice in South African gospel singing. This style of musical delivery will be explored more explicitly and in detail in chapter 6 of this work.

13. See "South African Mayor Defends Virgin Scholarships for Students." http://www.bbc.com/news/world-africa-35403501 (accessed on January 25, 2016).

Chapter 4

"We are a family"—Musical Space as Social Space of Communal Action

My work with the Siphithemba Choir went beyond the documentation of their songs and performances to extramusical contexts, whose environments provided me opportunities to immerse myself in their world so as to observe their processes of musical composition and performance, but also to appreciate how the spirituality of their music as a communal event is translated in their interactions with one another and with the larger society. Siphithemba Choir's membership consists of HIV-positive young men and women who have lost loved their ones—significant others, brothers, sisters, and friends—to the virus. Many have other family members living with the virus. They bring their personal experiences to the ensemble, and together they articulate and overlay them into a unique community ethos. As they struggle with the virus, they provide support to one another, both within the context of musical performance and in extramusical environments. They function as surrogate family to each other as they deal with the exigencies of the virus, including sickness, societal stigma, and joblessness. They even provide financial support to one another when necessary. Hence in this chapter, I examine the extramusical aspects of the choir in terms of their membership, organizing, and mutual social and economic support. Drawing upon my conversations with choir members, I argue that the sense of community that characterizes the choir's organization and functionality is rooted in the Zulu and Nguni social philosophy of *ubuntu,* a philosophy that extolls human interdependency; the interconnectedness of person to person, and the well-being of humans to the well-being of their environment. This social philosophy has spiritual, social, economic, and health ramifications for individuals who must live as members of a community.

In the course of this research, the concept and public discourse on *ubuntu* were very much in evidence. *Ubuntu* is often invoked in conversations related to post-apartheid reconciliation efforts, and to HIV/AIDS, especially with regard to stigma, honesty in relationships, and the empowerment of those who live on social and economic margins. During my fieldwork, I had engaging conversations with Zulu scholars and cultural activists. I conversed with members of the Siphithemba Choir to see to what extent this thought impacts their activities. My discourse on *ubuntu* philosophy in this work is drawn from these dialogues and reading, hence I use it to interpret the choir's organizing, and how they function as a community of mutual support to one another. Ultimately, the communal nature of their organizing and relationship found expression in the nature and process of musical production, both in terms of composition and performance as will be demonstrated later in this work.

Ubuntu is an existential natural philosophy of humanness with social and spiritual configurations. The meaning of the concept is succinctly captured in the Zulu expression *Umuntu ungumuntu ngabantu* (a person is a person because of other persons). According to Mathole Motshekga, a philosopher and founding director of the Kara Heritage Institute in Mamelodi, Pretoria, *ubuntu* explains a sense of community, wherein one's humanity is caught up in the humanity of others, irrespective of their race, gender, economic, or political class (SABC 2007)—and here, we can add, irrespective of their human immuno-viral status.

As a social philosophy, *ubuntu* establishes the mutual interdependency of human beings in the community, without the recognition of which the society easily dissolves into a state of chaos (Samkange and Samkange 1980). Nevertheless, late Thokozani Nene, a well-respected voice on Zulu culture and former host of cultural program on the Zulu Radio Ukhozi, cautioned against hellenizing this concept by construing it as a golden-rule form of social philosophy. According to him, "every individual person has *ubuntu* that is also tied to another person's *ubuntu*" (2006). In other words, every individual action has potential affect on another's life and that of the community. According to Nene, one potentially upsets the collective humanity by hurting another's *ubuntu,* but he or she also does as much harm when he or she hurts himself or herself by indulging, for example, in behaviors that undermine one's well-being. Both Thokozani Nene and Mathole Motshekga agree that *ubuntu* as a cosmological and spiritual configuration of human intersubjective mode of existence is sustainable only via a continued reevaluation and strengthening of each person's *ubuntu.*

Ubuntu is also a philosophy of well-being. In Zulu, *ukuphila* 'wellbeing' is tied to *ubuntu* inasmuch as the collective humanity of the community consists in the well-being of every member of the community. To achieve collective well-being, ferocious individual competitiveness is mitigated through communal ownership of land, which enables all members of the community to have a means to earn a living and to raise a family. In a radio program hosted by Xolani Gwala on SAFM, Mathole Motshekga explained:

> You cannot enjoy *ubuntu* if you have no access to land, if you have no access to economic development. So *ubuntu* must be the fountainhead of social and economic rights. So when we talk about moral regeneration, we must talk about uplifting people from their subhuman conditions and giving them access to socioeconomic rights, which would include access to land [and] participation in the economy.

But, the sense of community and collective well-being does not necessarily guarantee the continued safeguard and sustainability of *ubuntu.* Nene explained that as a people, the Zulu understand that the flow in the humanity of the community can easily be threatened by unforeseen states of economic, social, political, and even environmental emergencies; or still by personal avarice and ego (2006). Such emergent situations must be addressed by collective effort through the process of *indaba.*

Indaba in IsiZulu means 'meeting, consultative forum, dialogue.' It refers to the process in which competing or complementing parties engage to resolve or to prevent emergent crises in the community. It provides a means of continuously evaluating the conditions that affect the community to ensure the sustenance of *ubuntu* through a collective *ukuphila.*

The indigenous philosophy of *ubuntu* was revived by the exponents of Black Theology and the Black Consciousness Movement at the height of the antiapartheid movement in the 1970s and the 1980s as means to give their movements a local meaning. In the 1990s, Archbishop Desmond Tutu, the champion of the post-apartheid reconciliation efforts, further adapted the philosophy as an ideology to bring about reconciliation and harmony among South Africa's racial and ethnic groups. Under the reconciliation project, "the ethical values of *ubuntu* include respect for others, helpfulness, community, sharing, caring, trust and unselfishness"; under these projects, "*ubuntu* underscores the importance of agreement or consensus, and gives priority to the well-being of the community as a whole" (New World Encyclopedia 2008.)

From the 1960s, the indigenous Nguni social philosophy of *ubuntu* began to be articulated in modern intellectual activities, namely in Black Theology, and the Black Consciousness Movement. Black Theology (also called contextual theology) emphasized the merging of action with words in the liberation movement. It was also partly inspired by Latin American liberation theology, which taught that Christianity could not be divorced from life as a whole. The core tenet of this theology is that the gospel is a spiritual message with practical implications in the here and now of human life, and that Jesus' message of freedom from bondage has relevance in temporal as well as spiritual life (Gutierrez 1973).

South African Black Theology also draws from that which found its articulation in the work of African American theologian James Cone in the 1960s, which sought to give Black Nationalism (particularly the Black Power Movement) a theological grounding (Cone 1969). The exponents of South African Black Theology did exactly the same by incorporating and merging forces with the Black Consciousness. As Father Lebamang Sebidi (1995),[1] a major proponent of Black Theology, stated:

> We regarded Black Theology as the theological manifestation of the concerns expressed by Black Consciousness. It was a theological expression of the basic concerns of Black Consciousness. They were feeding on each other. So that for us Black Consciousness concerns, were the concerns of God, of the church, of the basic ethical Christianity. They were taken up by us and we supported the movement with this kind of theological vehicle. Black Theology was Black Consciousness at prayer.

For Father Sebidi, the two were just sides of the same coin, and members of the two movements worked closely together and attended meetings together, voicing the same concerns in the same language. No wonder, then, that this merging of ideas caused Archbishop Tutu to construe Black Consciousness as "a theology of black identity" (Battle 1997: 81; Tutu 2004: ix).

There is, however, a fundamental difference between South American liberation theology and Black Theology. While the former takes a Marxist approach and emphasizes the oppressor–oppressed relationship, the latter deploys the Nguni philosophy of *ubuntu* for analysis of the same mode of relationship. In a paper delivered at the joint conference of the Interdenominational Association of African Ministers of Religion and the Association for the Educational and Cultural Development of the African People in Edendale, Natal, in 1971, Steve Biko summarized the philosophy of *ubuntu* in his thought thus:

> "We enjoy man for himself. We regard our living together not as an unfortunate mishap warranting endless competition among us but as a deliberate act of God to make us a community of brothers and sisters jointly involved in the quest for a composite answer to the varied problems of life. (Biko 1971 [2004]: 46)

Similarly, Archbishop Tutu, following Bonganjalo Goba, a major exponent of Black Theology, articulated the African sense of *ubuntu* as "corporate personality," the "idea of solidarity, a social consciousness[,] . . . a caring concern that seeks to embrace all, a love that suffers selflessly for others" (Tutu 1973: 21). The theologizing of *ubuntu* as a discourse within Black Theology found strongest expression in Tutu's voice by his insertion of the concept of *imago Dei* into the discourse. For Tutu, the fundamental factor in the formation of the human community is the recognition of oneself and other persons as created in the image of God, irrespective of our physical differences. It stresses that God created the human community as a mutually interdependent system, where everyone is born with potentials that must be realized in the context of others and God (Battle 1997: 44). Black Theology thus informed by *ubuntu,* advocates that every individual be helped, and not hindered, to realize his or her full human potentials. This theology seeks to protect the oppressed, the weakest, and most vulnerable. It teaches that every individual is creative and illustrious, and must have the chance to attain the self-worth and fulfillment that come with industry and productivity.

Unfortunately, apartheid deprived Black South Africans of education and the benefits of economic freedom that might have come with it. It is for this reason that Biko observed: "because of the tradition forced onto the country, the poor people shall always be Black people. It is not surprising, therefore, that Black people should wish to rid themselves of a system that locks up the wealth of the country in the hands of a few" (Biko 1972[2004]: 68). In the light of the realization that poor people needed to be economically emancipated, churches began to set up community-resource centers and self-help income-generating projects aimed at creating self-reliant and economically empowered Black communities. According to Father Simangaliso Mkhatshwa's testimony, many members of the Black Consciousness Movement were deeply involved in establishing the earliest of these projects in parishes.[2] The first of these projects was arguably that established by Steve Biko in his hometown, King Williamstown. In the late 1970s, under the leadership of Denis Hurley, Roman Catholic Archbishop of Durban, the Diakonia Council of Churches in Durban established several community-resource centers that operated self-help projects in townships around Durban. In the 1980s, Archbishop Hurley began redistributing church lands to Black communities to enable them to engage in meaningful and sustainable income-generating farming. In the course of this research I visited several of the self-help projects, including KwaMashu Community Resource Center, KwaMakutha Community Resource Center, St. Clement Home-Based Care Project, and Clermont Community Resource Center. All these projects—founded in the apartheid era, with the exception of St. Clement Home-Based Care Project—have made easy transitions to addressing HIV/AIDS in their communities. Almost all of them are running HIV/AIDS support groups and self-help projects such as gardening (see figure 4.1), woodworking, and beadworking. The pairing of HIV/AIDS projects with income-generating projects in these resource centers is predicated on understanding that AIDS and poverty have symbiotic effects in people's lives.

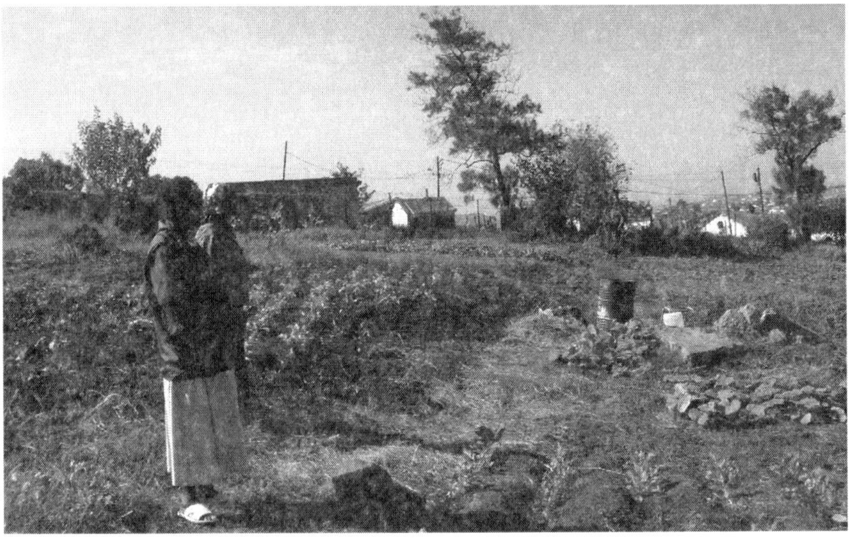

Figure 4.1 Self-help Gardening Project by the KwaMashu Community Resource Center.

Factsheet No. 52, published by the Pietermaritzburg Agency for Christian Social Awareness (August 2004) lists social and psychological indications that exacerbate the spread of the disease in South Africa. According to the factsheet, "52% of South Africans live below the poverty line." Their poor conditions of living and nutrition make them more vulnerable to infections, or if already HIV—positive, vulnerable to opportunistic infections as their immune systems weaken faster, compared with those who live in wealthy conditions. Poverty has also been linked to sexual behaviors that increase the risk of contracting HIV, such as prostitution and transactional sex.

Prolonged poverty can lead to depression and loss of hope, often culminating in risky and careless behaviors, such as drug use, alcoholism, and unprotected sex. All over South Africa, church institutions such as the Diakonia Council of Churches in Durban and the Pietermaritzburg Agency for Christian Social Awareness have been providing grassroots education and mobilization in the communities, encouraging people to participate in income-generating projects as a strategy for alleviating poverty. In the Durban area, Diakonia provides trainings for staff of the community-resource centers on how to run HIV/AIDS support groups and how to start and sustain income-generating projects.

The practical dimension of *ubuntu* in South African Black Theology is not restricted to establishing income-generating projects and community-resource centers. The *ubuntu* axiom that one's humanity is bound up with those of others has once again become a dominant perspective in the

HIV/AIDS discourse. From the viewpoint of the moral economy of HIV/AIDS, Nicoli Nattrass argues that the disease not only has deep social roots, but "challenges the very notion of what it means to be a society" (2004:189). In the light of this, Archbishop Ndungane of Cape Town remarks that "we have to become aware of our mutual entanglement, which must prompt us to care, to support, and to avoid the sin of stigmatization of those infected" (Ndungane 2003: 57–63). This form of "pragmatic solidarity" (Schmid 2006: 103) with people living with AIDS is required to stop the moralization of the disease—an attitude that has characterized responses from some church hierarchies. This understanding caused the churches to merge forces with the Treatment Action Campaign to mobilize the public in pressuring the South African government to change its policy and agree to provide treatment for people living with AIDS (de Gruchy and de Gruchy 2005: 235). The mission hospitals are among the first to roll out treatment for these people. In the Durban area, these institutions include the McCord Hospital of the Congregationalist Church and the Marianhill (Roman Catholic) Hospital. McCord is particularly of interest because of its role in giving birth to the Siphithemba Choir: it continued to provide treatment for members of the Sinikithemba Support Group and the choir. This action is predicated on the conviction that those who have HIV and AIDS can still live and be as productive as ordinary citizens; it dispels the fear of those who are infected. This attitude, as I show in this chapter, characterizes the resilience and hope that the Siphithemba choir members carry with them, both in their music and in their daily lives.

Black Consciousness and Black Theology emphasize the spiritual connectedness of human beings as embedded in the *ubuntu* discourse while giving it a theological interpretation, but they draw upon the collective-well-being aspect of the philosophy to emphasize the practical dimensions of the movement and theology.

SIPHITHEMBA CHOIR AND THE PRACTICE OF UBUNTU

In interviews, Mrs. Nonhlanhla Mhlongo, who founded the Sinikithemba Support Group and the Siphithemba Choir, emphasized the communal spirit and sense of family that characterized the operation of the group from its inception. The communal spirit and sense of family were particularly manifest on two levels. First, members looked out for one another to forestall the chances that members would sicken and die without getting the spiritual support they needed. In her words, "the group was like a family. They were supposed to come only on Tuesdays, but people will come on Monday to Friday because of family environment. . . . If a member doesn't show up, Siphokazi [pseudonym], she will say 'where is so and so?'" To strengthen their effort to look out for one another, the members of the support group divided into small groups according to their townships and areas of residences. These groups visited sick or bereaved members in their areas and provided them with the support of prayers and helping with housekeeping.

Second, when members began to generate incomes through their bead-work, other crafts, and concert tours, the support group created a trust fund, which, according to Mrs. Mhlongo, was designed to support the education and sustenance of deceased members' children and spouses.

On a follow-up conversation after a support-group meeting in her office, I asked Mrs. Mhlongo if these manifest senses of family and community could be interpreted as, or similar to, the Zulu sense of *ubuntu*. Her response was, "*yebo, baba* Austin [yes, father Austin], because *ubuntu* is all about community and how you take care of one another." The following dialogue ensued:

> *Q*. So does it mean that all members of the group are aware of these ways of organizing the support group as a practice of *ubuntu*?
>
> *A*. [Hesitatingly] Eh, *baba*, honestly, all I can tell you is that—. (At this point, Nqobile [pseudonym] from her desk where she was working on her beads, interjected in Zulu, reminding Mrs. Mhlongo how they had talked about it sometimes during their meetings, especially when some members had not shown up for funerals). Yes, we talked about it sometimes. Yes, they know about it.
>
> *Q*. But, by the way, this sounds like what church groups would do also. So one can also argue that you are just doing these things because of your Christian faith.
>
> *A*. Yes. It is also because we are Christians. But I think it is also more because that is how we do things as Zulu people, like if you go in the townships, or even in the rural areas, like where I come from, if you are a mother, and you prepare food for your family, but you see other children from the homestead, and their mother is not home, and they have nothing to eat, you also give them the food to eat; you share with them. So you can say that that is a Christian way of doing things, but that is also our culture as Zulu people.

Mrs. Mhlongo's insistence that the support group and choir's way of operating is as a result of who they are as Zulu people and therefore amounted to the practice of *ubuntu* was consistent with Nomusa Mpanza's statement: "I think it [the way they operated] has to do with us as Zulu people. Because there was another support group that was made of White people and some Indian people and coloureds people; and what they did was totally different from the way we operated." I had heard about this support group during my visits to McCord Hospital, but had not met any of its members. Monti Thomas, who coordinated the team of counselors at the Sinikithemba Clinic, explained that the group met infrequently, and did not have a cohesive structure like the Zulu group. Nomusa gave examples of members of the other support group not attending their group members' funerals, whereas the Zulu group attended the funerals of members from both groups.

Phumlani Kunene, conductor of the choir, gave an interpretation of *ubuntu* that was more global than the way other members spoke about it. He expanded the "community" beyond the support group and the choir to their communities in Durban and beyond—in South Africa, and even Africa. He explained that "anything you do to help anybody, anywhere is the same as *ubuntu. Ubuntu* just means that we have to work together all the time." His global perspective would become clearer to me as I analyzed the songs of the choir, many of which he had composed, either by himself, or together with other choir members.

Phakamile Shabane explained her understanding of *ubuntu* in relation to the choir thus:

> *Ubuntu* actually refers to the good actions or deeds that a particular someone do [*sic*] to the other to show how much he or she cares about him or her in that particular situation. Based on the history of the choir, there are things which happened or [are] still happening. To mention a few, to be on each other's back [i.e., to be supportive] when he or she is in a hard situation, to get someone a job if you are in an appropriate position. With the case of the choir members alone, there are a couple of things which we did or [are] still doing for each other.

Phakamile's explanation brings to mind the dimension of communal well-being that Dr. Mathole Motshekga describes above. It was partly the sense of communal well-being that had motivated Xolani Zulu to found the African Vision Shop (to be explored further), through which he provided employment for members who had no source of income. The same sense of wellbeing accounted for the transformation of the support group into an income-generating project when a member offered to teach others how to make beads. In effect, the members of the Siphithemba Choir showed clear understanding of what they did, and how they did it, as stemming from their background and worldview as Zulu. It is this worldview that informed their ability to function as a support group that provides spiritual and emotional support to members primarily through songs. But the operation of the choir became a source of income for members through their national and international tours. Members continue to make bead projects, which they market overseas, especially in the United States. They also accumulated income from sale of the CD recordings. It is the same worldview that informs their commitment to bringing the message of hope to their local community through their songs, and to educate them on the need for disease prevention and treatment.

Choir Structure

Perhaps it is in the organization of the choir that the culture of *ubuntu* is most evident. The membership of the choir in the course of this study stood at about twenty, though I met only about fifteen during most of my work with the group. Some were absent during the period, mostly because of ill health. Those who performed regularly during my extended period of work with the group between 2006 and 2007 included Phumlani Kunene as choir director; Sizwe Ndlela as accompanist and assistant director; Xolani Zulu, who sings baritone and plays the bass and drum sets; Phakamile Shabane, Wicky Shabane, and Nokuthula, sopranos; Zinhle Thabetha, Ncamisile Yengwa, Nelly, and Nozipho, altos; Sizile and Nomusa Mpanza, countertenors; and Super and Bheki, baritones. Most of these and a few old members who weren't there during my extended stay were also present when they joined me for a concert at the Emmanuel Cathedral in Durban with the Williams College Chamber Choir in 2012.

At the extended period of research, the choir was in the process of registering as an incorporated nonprofit organization. Phumlani Kunene remained its conductor. Sizwe Ndlela functioned as his assistant, and Xolani helped with administrative matters. Other designated posts included the finance committee, consisting of Xolani, Wicky, and Zinhle; and the costumes committee, consisting of Xolani, Nokuthula, Wicky, and Nomusa.

With regard to the music leadership, any member who feels strong enough to lead can take up the leadership in the absence of Phumlani and Sizwe. I witnessed Xolani, Zinhle, Super, and Phakamile rehearse the choir with ease on occasions when neither Phumlani nor Sizwe were present. Whenever any of these members assumed the leadership role, other members usually took their singing positions to ensure that the other's leadership for the day would be a success. A sense of community devoid of unnecessary competition formed part of the inner ethos of Siphithemba.

In his *ubuntu* theology, Archbishop Desmond Tutu reiterates the fact that an unnecessarily high degree of competition breeds selfishness and creates the greatest discrepancy of "incommensurate difference," which negates God's creative purpose of mutual interdependence (Battle 1997: 41). Thus, in the choir, there is an understanding that the failure of one member is the failure of all, just as the success of one proves a point of success for the others. Just as all are individually determined to live in the face of the disease, so are they determined collectively to see to the survival of the group, the one space that has proven to be a bastion of hope and the epitome of a positive experience for each of them.

Siphithemba was divided into subgroups, including two rehearsal sections dedicated to traditional song and gospel music, respectively. According to Phumlani, the subgroups were created because most members were now employed and busy during the week. The choir could rehearse together for less than two hours a week, on Sunday afternoons. Some people, however, were free on certain days of the week, so they come together to rehearse in groups of three or four, as the case may be. The weekday rehearsals were used mainly to compose and learn new songs, which were then learned by the large group on Sunday afternoons. Dance movements are choreographed and integrated with the songs during Sunday rehearsals. In this way, songs were learned faster, and the repertory continued to grow. As Phumlani's assistant, Sizwe rehearsed most of the subgroups. Since he has strong keyboard skills, he worked as the ensemble's accompanist, and he oversaw the choir's instruments and other sound equipment.

A Community of Mutual Support

Another indicator of a strong sense of community that characterized the inner operations of Siphithemba is that members were always present for one another in good times and in bad, in celebration of life and death. At one of the choir's rehearsal at Umlazi, a Poptec film crew from Maine was to record the choir for a film documentary. At the end of the film-shooting session, Sizwe and Phumlani approached me to invite me to an *umsebenzi*[3] that was to take place at Sizwe's family home in Nyoni, a rural town about 130 kilometers north of Durban. The event marked the unveiling of the tombs of Sizwe's grandmother and two siblings, who had all died less than two years before. It was a two-day event, which started on Friday with the ritual slaughtering of three goats, one for each of the diseased, and culminating in the slaughtering of, and feasting on, two cows on Saturday, in which all the members of the Ndlela family and their neighbors and friends participated.

Phumlani pleaded with me to come with them on Friday, but I declined because I would have to come back to Durban on Saturday morning to preside at the Sacrament of Reconciliations at the Emmanuel Cathedral—an event I nevertheless forgot about and missed because I zoomed off to Nyoni the next morning, out of curiosity to be present to witness the event. Upon reflection, I wondered if Phumlani had been coaxing me to come on Friday so that I could witness the entire ritual, or so I could provide needed extra transport. We agreed finally that I would go with Phakamile, Nomusa, and Nokthula on Saturday morning.

Some of the men, including Phumlani and Super, went with Sizwe on Friday afternoon to help with preparing the animals and the meat and to do the chores in preparation for Saturday. At the event, most of us mixed with Sizwe's family by helping with chores. I even got the duty of *ukuqoba,* the cutting of the broiled meat, "a man's job, if you are the man with other women" according to Phakamile. Later on, Phakamile and Nomusa told me that Sizwe's family and people in attendance were full of praise for Sizwe, because of his friends who were present and helping in the chores. They even commented on my presence, and how I conveyed a sense that I felt at home among them, because I did not shy away from taking up roles in the ceremony. In effect, I argue that the sense of family that the choir shares not only helped shape the social identity of the group, but helped members renegotiate their relationships with their families, who are now more open toward them, by appreciating their human capabilities in spite their HIV status.

The act of being there for one another is useful as a support mechanism for members when they have had to disclose their status to their families. An example is the case of two sisters, Wicky and Phakamile, when the entire choir rallied round them by traveling with them to their rural home in Highflats, as they disclosed their status to their family. Status disclosure has been recognized in the HIV/AIDS discourse as about the most difficult thing with which people living with the virus have to deal. The intent to disclose brings anxiety because of unforeseeable consequences of rejection and stigmatization. For this reason, people living with AIDS are encouraged to receive counseling before disclosure, and often are encouraged to find a "safe space and right moment" (Ntsimane 2006: 12–13) for doing so. For the members of Siphithemba Choir, their safe space and right moment is particularly in the

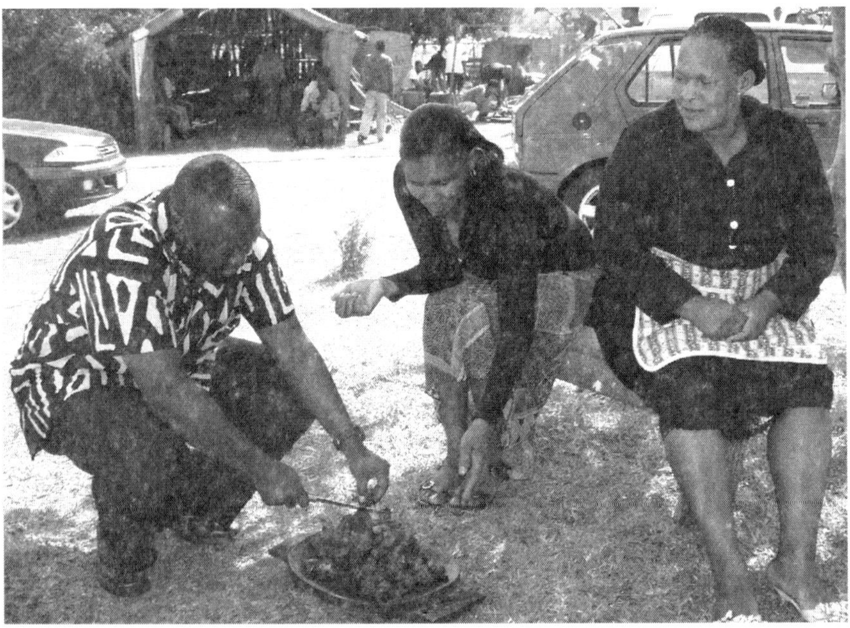

Figure 4.2 Author participates in *umsebenzi* at Nyoni.

presence of choir members, who function as surrogate family to one another, and are in the struggle together.

XOLANI AND THE AFRICAN VISION SHOP

Xolani's African Vision Shop, which has now closed at the time of the revision of this manuscript, was located in Durban's City Business District on West Street, about two blocks from the beaches of the Indian Ocean. It was a fashion shop that designed "traditional" Southern African dresses. On my first visit, the shop appeared to be a big business in the making. It was simply a show room, because one could see all the different fashion designs through the transparent screen walls facing the street. Inside, on the wall, and well arranged all over the floor area were several more designs of Xhosa women's outfits, some men's suits made from Basotho *seshoeshoe* 'wax print' material, and a host of male, female, and unisex T-shirts with the heads of Steve Biko, Nelson Mandela, Martin Luther King Jr., Rita Marley, and other Black leaders.

On the east wall of the shop was an old couch with a coffee table against it. On the table was a photo album full of women's pictures, including those of a White American girl who had modeled some designs from the shop. On a cashier's counter on the opposite wall were littered assorted beadworks, some of which were hanging on the wall. Some, Xolani made me understand, had been made by members of the Sinikithemba Support Group who were still making a living from the skills they had acquired at McCord Hospital. The showroom section of the shop, which faces West Street, was separated from the inner chamber by the cashier's counter on the west wall and a dwarf wall on the east wall next to the couch. In the inner chamber were three electric sewing machines. A personal laptop computer rested on the design table, positioned against dwarf shelves that contained textiles that were yet to be cut into designs. There was busy production activity going on, with some women—including Wicky and Nokuthula, Siphithemba Choir members—and a man named Dipa at work on the machines, with whom I would later become acquainted.

During a subsequent interview, Xolani explained that he had quit his job at a steel company to start the African Vision Shop in October 2004. His purpose was to manage his time more freely, so as to be able to participate fully in the choir's activities and tours. His decision was informed by the fact that other choir members, who, after their health had improved from treatment at McCord Hospital, and finding new employment opportunities, had quit the ensemble because their new jobs did not permit them to tour with the choir. Tours had become sources of income for the choir members, especially the tours overseas, but the tours occurred only once or twice a year; members therefore had to have some regular income during the rest of the year. Xolani chose his participation in the choir over his steel-company job because of his desire to continue to sing, but most especially because he had a capital base to build upon. As a person with entrepreneurial skill, he could set up a successful business.

I discussed in chapter 2 that initially most members of the Sinikithemba Support Group were not gainfully employed (some for lack of skills), or had lost their jobs. Whereas some support-group members who received HIV counseling training at McCord were retained at the hospital, including three members of Siphithemba Choir (Sizile, Ncamisile, and Nomusa), many were still jobless when the ensemble separated from McCord. Xolani brought two of them to work with him in the shop, so they too could earn income. He did not have experience in fashion designing, so he simply ran the business management part of the shop. Wicky, a choir member who worked with him, was the only one from the Sinikithemba Support Group who had been trained in sewing. Xolani brought Dipa, who was versatile in designing, to work with them. The shop thus functioned as a center for production and training. Here again I must point out the sense of community that guided the Siphithemba members' efforts to work together, and their characteristic sense of *ubuntu,* which made them look out for one another's well-being. At the time of this study, Xolani was earning a certificate course in fashion designing and management at the Durban University of Technology to enhance his managerial skills.

Since the African Vision Shop's employees were members of the Siphithemba Choir, they helped design some of the choir's costumes. But in the main, Xolani's vision was to collect and produce as many African textiles and fashion styles as possible. The shop already had a few Nigerian and Congolese dresses in it; this area was not yet extensive, but the vision had a sense of pan-Africanism—which probably explains the name *African Vision Shop.* I shall not dwell on this here, but I point out later, in my analyses of Siphithemba music, that pan-African vision and consciousness is not unique to Xolani: in singing about HIV/AIDS, Siphithemba members claim to join their struggle to that of the rest of Africa.

THE POWER OF POSITIVE LIVING

"Living positively," or "positive living," is an expression that one hears often in HIV/AIDS support-group meetings in South Africa. It is a dominant theme in HIV discourse and AIDS counseling, which conveys the concept of having a positive emotional and spiritual attitude toward and about the reality of the disease. The choir conductor, Phumlani Kunene, describes it as a form of spiritual disposition because "I must thank God everyday for keeping me alive. Many people have died, you know. But we are alive, and many of us have jobs or doing one thing or the other and taking care of ourselves and our kids. Some people didn't think before that we could do that." In another interview for a film documentary by Hainsworth (2005), he represented his act of positive living thus:

Each day that comes, I enjoy it.
The day that comes, I salute it.
The day that comes, I thank God.
The day that comes, I respect God.
So I will keep on living a very positive life,
And I will keep on saying things to the people,
To live positively.[4]

Positive living is also used by people living with AIDS, AIDS activists, and counselors in places other than South Africa. In an interview with Gregory Barz, Kasule described "positive living" as "a way of changing your attitude towards whatever has happened to you and going clockwise. You can't go anti-clockwise. Looking at your chances, looking at your opportunities, and looking at how best you can start from there" (Barz 2006: 52).

Among members of the Siphithemba Choir, stories abound about the burdens of being HIV-positive. Nomusa's partner, with whom she had had two daughters, denied having had anything to do with her infection and accused her of infidelity. Ncamisile's boyfriend and father of her daughter walked out of her life and denied having had anything to do with her positive status; for a while, her family members avoided her daughter, even after she had been determined to be HIV-negative. For these people, the will to live entails avoiding dwelling with perpetual regret about what has happened to them. The idea of positive living can be defined as the psychology of living with the reality of AIDS. For the Siphithemba choir and support group, it is an attitude that is relevant for both the infected and the noninfected. Its efficacy lies in living above denial, knowing one's status, and avoiding the stress and depression that stems from anxiety and uncertainty, seeking appropriate help in the form of treatment, networking with people who share the experience of being infected or affected, and striving to stay HIV-negative. For Siphithemba members, this means finding ways to lead a meaningful life and contributing to one's family and community, rather than dwelling on regrets and self-pity. It is by this attitude to life that people living with AIDS can reaffirm their humanity, which has been challenged by the disease, social stigma, and rejection by friends and family.

It is the power of positive living that informed Mrs. Mhlongo's position when she asserted, "What we are trying to inculcate to people is that they have to work and not beg. Because of their status, they shouldn't go around begging; instead, they should give something in return." Thus, for the support group and the choir, positive living consists of finding fulfillment in and through work. It is for this reason that the microeconomic and skills-acquisition project was developed. Siphithemba members have continued to maintain this attitude in different ways, exemplified, for example, in Xolani's African Vision Shop: some of them have gone back to school; others have gone on to receive further training. Presently, almost all are employed gainfully as AIDS counselors in hospitals, in HIV/AIDS/STI research projects, in textile and fashion designing, or in beadwork and productions.

The choir and support group are social network systems. In addition to making music, members monitor one another and provide support to one another as they deal with the experience of being HIV-positive. The gatherings of the ensemble, its rehearsals, and its tours and performances, comprised recreational activities for members as a group who share common experiences of rejection and social stigma.

Speaking of recreation, this includes exercise, which has been recognized as a key component of positive living (O'Loughlin 2008). While attending several HIV/AIDS support-group meetings and workshops, I saw constant reminders to people living with AIDS to keep fit and strengthen their immune system through regular exercise. When I asked the choir how they do this, Phumlani quickly responded, "by dancing." According to him, Zulu

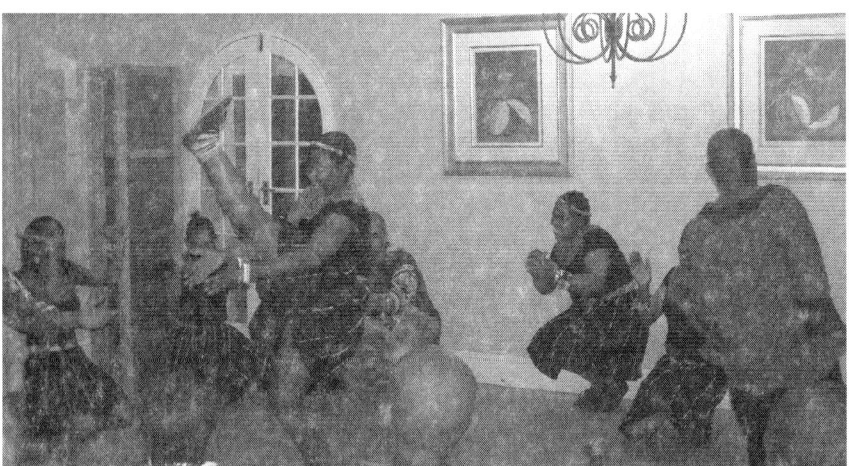

Figure 4.3 Ncamisile demonstrates the *ukusina* dance.

traditional songs, with their accompanying vigorous dance movements and heavy foot-stamping, provide weekly exercise for members who would not otherwise have an opportunity to exercise because of their schedules and environments. Thus, making music plays several roles for the choir members in their struggle with HIV/AIDS: as income-generating enterprise, talent expression, social network, and outlet for physical exercise.

In effect, musical performance paired with dance, in addition to helping to strengthen the health of individual members, equally strengthens the collective health of the group including their existence as a social entity.

SUMMARY AND CONCLUSION

Throughout my work with the Siphithemba Choir, its members emphasized for me how being in the choir comprised a home and family for them. This sense of being with family in the choir is even shared sometimes by relatives of choir members. For example on one Sunday afternoon, the choir broke up the rehearsal earlier than normal so all the members could visit Super's home in Umlazi township and join his family in a celebration. Super's mother had had a thanksgiving service at the church for reason that was not explained to me. The choir did some performances of songs and dance in the family living room, in which Super's mother and siblings also participated. Super's mother at the end spoke and thanked the choir for taking care of her son. She got very emotional when she explained how she had worried about Super who, since discovering his HIV-positive status had shifted from his former routine social activities and relationships in the neighborhood to a seeming isolated lifestyle. Yet she marveled at how much her son had matured since then, looking much healthier, and being a lot focused on his work and studies. At this point Super was studying computer programing in Durban. In his mother's words, "now I know that he has a family that is taking good care of him."

Speaking of the choir's musical space as a space of communal social action therefore, I tried in this chapter to show the various levels at which their sense of community is manifest—namely as mutual support of one another in coping with the stress that comes with being HIV-positive; as support mechanism when a member has had to make disclosure of their status to their immediate family; their helping one another in finding jobs or acquiring occupational trainings for the purpose of becoming economically self-reliant. Most especially, their music comprise a means of engaging in positive living given that singing and dancing afforded them the benefit of spiritual, emotional, and physical health as they deal with a disease whose cure is still far removed.

NOTES

1. Information is from the Sinomlando Project of the UKZN Theology Department, courtesy of the Alan Paton Center and Struggles Archive, UKZN, Pietermaritzburg.

2. This information is from the Sinomlando Project of the UKZN Theology Department 1995, courtesy of the Alan Paton Center and Struggles Archive, UKZN, Pietermaritzburg.

3. *Umsebenzi* means 'work' in Zulu, but can refer to major ritual events in the family, especially the unveiling of tombs, during which goats and cows are slaughtered and prepared for the feasting.

4. I purposefully put this quote in a block to show the rhyme and rhythm (see Hainsworth 2005).

Chapter 5

"We Sing with One Mind and Purpose"

Expressing Spirituality and Sociocultural Experience

At the end of the collaborative concert with the Siphithemba Choir at the Emmanuel Cathedral, Durban in January 2012, one of my Williams College students approached a few Siphithemba members who were exchanging pleasantries with me and expressed astonishment at how few voices there are in the Siphithemba Choir but yet they carried such volume that almost surpassed that of the Williams Choir of more than thirty voices. One of the members, Phakamile Shabane, who was standing with me, responded, "Well, we sing with one mind and purpose." As casual as her response came across however, it touched on the actual musical dimension of Siphithemba's history and organization, which I argued in the forgone chapter as characterized by the sense of family, wherein the choir members work and overlay their experiences together in their struggle with HIV/AIDS. Their success thus hinges on their ability to draw upon that experience and quest for well-being, which spurs them on and engenders their resilience, creativity, and determination to beat the perceived odds of being HIV-positive. It also points to the purposefulness of their songs and music making, which may be appreciated especially by exploring their musical choices, and the messages and meanings of their songs.

By exploring their musical choices and the meanings embedded in their songs in this chapter, some historical significance comes to light: namely their music recalls the creative precedents that have been witnessed in the history of South African choral tradition, especially in the deployment of the genre of struggle, a genre now being taken into the context of the HIV/AIDS experience. To make this extant enough, I periodically juxtapose their songs with other historical compositions ranging from the songs of the Zulu Nazarite Church, to those of eclectic composers such as Enoch Sontonga and John Knox Bokwe. Thus I argue that while the Siphithemba songs index historical song examples, the choir speaks to its members' experience; to their local community; Africa; and the world as a concentric audience, by reiterating the message of hope, reinterpreting the struggle experience, and advocating for behavior change.

MUSICAL GENRE: GOSPEL VERSUS TRADITIONAL

My use of the words *gospel* and *traditional* in this work reflects the word choice of my research collaborators. I understand the problematic implications of the word *tradition* in the context of ethnography, but as I have argued from the beginning, following in the footsteps of scholars who have come before me, the views of local participants in this research and the meanings they make of the concepts they employ to explain their activities are as important as any effort at exegetical analysis of the word.

The term *traditional* in local musical contexts in Africa is complex. In the work of J. H. Kwabena Nketia, the use of the phrase *traditional music,* especially in Ghana, suggests permanence and exclusiveness in "unadulterated form outside the adopted Western institution" (1974: 16). This description is predicated on an understanding that traditional musicians and their music were excluded from the church and educational institutions, which comprised the direct source of Western influence. They are preserved and flourish within the space of the "traditional political, social and cultural institutions that support them" and which have endured in the presence of Christianity, Western cultural institutions, and colonialism (1974: 16). A similar sense is implied in the categorization used by the Igbo Service Division of the Imo Broadcasting Service in Owerri, Nigeria, to describe the genres of secular music that were heard on medium-wave broadcasts from the 1970s through 1990s. *Egwu odinala,* literally 'music that is on the ground,' is a set of genres that have indigenous origins. The concept often implies some sense of permanence and exclusivity to traditional political and social institutions. *Egwu agwalagwa,* literally 'mix-match music,' is so called because it combines elements of indigenous and Western music. This category is indeed popular music, and it is further subdivided into *egwu agba ochie* 'old-time music' and *egwu agba ohuru* 'contemporary music'; the subdivision is based on a historical timeline, in which independence, achieved in 1960, serves as a marker between the latter and the former. The categorizations made by Nketia and the Igbo service division of the Imo Broadcasting Service tended to construe the so-called indigenous or traditional music as insulated from the wave of colonialism, modernity, and the flow of information between the urban and rural, as has been argued by Karin Barber (1997).

In contrast, Carol A. Muller observes that what is described as traditional in the South African experience does not imply that which never changes; instead, she observes that some musics "labeled 'traditional' in the 1990s were music that sounded quite different from its ancestral forms performed earlier in the twentieth century" (2004: 5). These include popular genres, such as the Zulu *maskanda*, which she calls hybrid forms of traditional performances that were created in urban environments, drawing on elements of European music.

These categorizations, whether in the case of Igbo of Eastern Nigeria, Ghana, or South Africa, are all referents of music genres other than the choral-music tradition shaped by mission Christianity. In choral-music performance, however, there exists a disparity between such institutional domains as the national choral festival and noninstitutional domains, like the everyday choral activity that one might experience in the townships or in the rural areas in the use of the term *traditional.*

In the course of my work in South Africa, I learned that musicians, choral conductors, and organizers of choral-music festivals and competitions are careful not to bedevil their activities with the complex exigencies of the word *traditional.* Several choral competitions at local and national levels—including the grandest, the National Choir Festival, sponsored by two of South Africa's biggest corporate entities, The Old Mutual and Telcom—now avoid the use of the term in their categories. The competitions usually involve three selected categories, including "Western songs," "African songs," and "indigenous African songs" (National Finals Programme 2006).[1] "Western songs" are drawn from cantatas and oratorios of Western classical composers, especially Mozart and Handel. "African songs" are formally composed art music, which can be written by institutionally trained musicians or amateur composers; they can be religious or secular in their textual content, but they are set in indigenous languages. The "indigenous" category, in contrast, is drawn from, or at least is based on, folk-music formularies, transmitted orally and not written down. At the festivals that I witnessed, except in church music festivals, choirs tend to dress up in what they consider traditional attire: animal skin and beads for the Zulu; *seshoeshoe* 'wax print' materials for the Basotho, Batswana, and Bapedi; and colorful stripped calico materials for the Xhosa. The performance of this category of songs usually integrates indigenous dances, particularly the *ngoma* dance, in the case of the Zulu choirs.

Dr. Joshua Rhadebe, the veteran conductor of the Pietermaritzburg Choral Society, interviewed in Pietermaritzburg said the designation of the three categories does not appear to be an attempt to avoid the academic exigencies of the concept of "tradition." Momgi Mzobe and Sibusiso Mkhulusi, conductors of the African Chorus and Joy of Africa Chorus respectively, agree. For Mkhulusi, "The 'African songs' category is to encourage composers to look into these old ones, and maybe they can learn something from there when they compose the modern songs." In other words, the indigenous categories, which appear to have been a much later addition to the categories, are designed to preserve the folk and indigenous forms, which in turn would inform and shape the styles of modern art music compositions and performance.

So why do I chose then to use the word *traditional*? Where did it come from? While attending several choir rehearsals in townships, churches, and hospitals, I heard choristers and conductors use the expression *traditional song* often to refer to specific types of music, which correspond to the "indigenous" category described above. Generally, these include songs with Zulu folk and cultural themes. They are not formally composed: their form is usually call-and-response, with repetitive refrains, and they are usually paired with dance. Thus, although in official documents of regional and national choral festivals and competitions, organizers avoid the use of the term, choristers and choirmasters have a propensity to refer to this category of songs as traditional. Similarly, Siphithemba uses the term *traditional* to refer to a similar category of songs in its repertory, as opposed to its primary repertoires, which comprise recognizably religious music embedded with Christian gospel messages, such as the praise of God, proclamation of the word, and eschatology.

WHY TRADITIONAL MUSIC?

I have argued somewhere else (see Okigbo 2014) that members of the Siphithemba Choir do not see any inherent contradictions between African cultural values, ideals, and symbols and the Christian gospel message. From the members' perspective, the incorporation of African traditional songs serves as a powerful tool in transmitting their gospel of hope using a form that is recognizable to their local communities. They do not just randomly sing traditional tunes: they consciously select songs that they judge to be relevant to the message they want to spread about HIV/AIDS.

On another level, I wish to put this in the context of the African cosmology that blurs the boundaries between the transcendent and the mundane. This is owing to a form of African metaphysics that juxtaposes the spiritual and physical worlds in an interconnected mode of existence (Mbiti 1970). Among the Igbo of southeastern Nigeria, *chi* and the ancestors are believed to involve themselves in the affairs of individuals and the community in general. Whereas every individual and every community has its *chi*, *chi* permeates the cosmic order of the Igbo in such a manner that one's well-being is dependent on the mode of existence within the interconnected world of spirits and humans. Every individual's actions in trade, agriculture, marriage, birth, and death, serve either to strengthen that mode of relationship, succinctly captured in the concept of *omenala* (customs, traditions, morals, spirituality, and industry), or to disrupt that relationship, in the form of *imerụala* 'to defile the land.'

Among the Basotho of Southern Africa, a similar metaphysics is seen in the economy of *bophelo* 'well-being,' in which the individual (*motho*) and his/her activities and well-being are at the heart of a relationship between him/her, the family (*lelapa*), the village (*motse*), the land (*naha)*, spirituality (*borapeli*), and the earth (*lefatse*), set in a sociospatial configuration.[2]

Among the Zulu, the concept of *ubuntu* is more than just a social philosophy of communality: it is a cosmic spirituality, which is either realized or disrupted by the way a person relates to another and to the state of things around him or her. It is so strong that when a person says that someone is hurting his or her *ubuntu*, it would also mean that one is actually disrupting his relationship with the cosmic order. Among the Igbo, this amounts to *imeruala;* and among the Basotho, it comprises a disruption of the individual's *bophelo.*

What I am trying to show here is the basis of an African worldview that holds the worlds of the sacred and the secular in an interconnected dynamism (Henderson 1995: 55). Conversion to Christianity, colonialism, and modern forms of secular state formations have not succeeded in upsetting this worldview in any significant way in people's day-to-day lives in many African societies, including the Zulu.

The blurring boundaries between the sacred and the secular are particularly evident in the involvement of churches in political and social affairs. In South Africa, church spaces have been used for political meetings and rallies. At the heart of this church involvement is the understanding that a spirituality of salvation has meaning and relevance in the lives of a people when it seeks to improve their economic, social, and political well-being, aspects of life that are constantly violated by an oppressive system.

The African worldview that blurs the boundary between the sacred and the secular is strongly evident in choral music in South Africa, especially in forms of resistance to oppression in the church and in the state. Some of the contents of Zulu Nazarite Church hymnody, for instance, are adaptations of Zulu folksongs, meshed with images of Zulu cosmology, kinship lineages, and Zulu warriors. Consider the parallel between the *ihubo* of the Buthelezi family, attributed to Ngqengelele (a greatgrandfather of Mangosuthu Buthelezi, the present chief of the Buthelezi family) and the Nazarite hymn number 173, "Sindedele Singene," by Isaiah Shembe[3]:

The Buthelezi *Ihubo*

We were cast away
From our father Shenge's place of olden time

What ails you, people?
Do you not know we were founded in olden days?
Now we are seated near the doorway.

Nazarite Hymn No. 173
Let us come in to worship Jehovah
We were shut out, but now the gates are open.
Let them in.
See! Here are the Zulus
Descendants of Dingana, and of Senzagkhona

The Buthelezi family has seen a series of feuds with other chiefs under the Zulu monarch for centuries. These feuds sometimes resulted in the loss of the family's close relationship with the reigning king; but later these relationships have always been restored. Ngqengelele's song is therefore a narration of this experience. The "doorway" in the song is a sign of close relationship to the king, because as a major adviser and probably as prime minister, the chief has the power to let people in or shut them out of the royal palace. Clearly, Isaiah Shembe used the technique of textual alteration to adapt the traditional song to a church hymn and thereby shift the context of the song and reinterpret the meaning to fit with Zulu experience of racial discrimination in the mission church. In their new worship space in the independent church, the people are now free, not only to worship according to their own cultural ideals and spirituality, but also to be their own leaders. The reference to Dingane and Senzagkhona makes the context and meaning of the song relevant to the Zulu people instead of simply the Buthelezi family. Similarly, church songs were appropriated for purposes of engaging resistance in the political arena prior to and during the apartheid era (Dargie 1997: 322–324; Detterbeck 2002: 147–150).

Traditional songs have always been part of the Siphithemba repertory. Some of the choir's most commonly performed repertoires in this genre include "Isiyalo" (Advice), "Ikhalaphi?" (From Whence the Cry?), and "Ibonakana nganina?" (How Does She Show She Loves Him?). Others are "Hamba, Lulu" (Go, Lulu), "Mama ndiyagoduga mgomso" (Mama, I'm Going Home Tomorrow), and "Seliyaduma" (It's Thundering).

In my conversations with Phumlani (the choir conductor) and other members of the choir, three reasons for their decision to incorporate traditional songs became apparent. According to Phumlani, "these traditional songs have a way of making people want to dance. So we really wanted to sing something that they understand, because they already know the meaning and what we are singing." Xolani Zulu provided a similar explanation. In other words, the choir members are concerned about getting their message across to their local audience, and so the best medium to that effect is a musical idiom that is recognizable to their local community.

During an interview, Xolani made the point that "we preach the gospel and give hope through our music." Asked how he sees the consistency of incorporating traditional songs with preaching the gospel, he responded, "because they are part of who we are as African people. I think it's okay: we can still praise God with traditional music, because we're doing good work with it." I had hinted on Phumlani's and Nomusa's explanation that the choir's decision to perform traditional songs was to provide more opportunities for dance. According to Nomusa, this was also a way to project their distinctive African identity in the context of performance. It appears therefore that there is at least an implicit consensus to the effect that the performance of traditional songs does not negate the Christian outlook of the ensemble, or the Christian principles of the McCord Hospital: rather, traditional songs add to the choir's versatility, and comprise part of the appropriate medium of speaking to South African audiences in recognizable form. Also, performing traditional songs helps project a distinctive African identity to foreign audiences. The need to connect with local audiences and project an African identity to foreign audiences also informed the choir's use of traditional Zulu dresses as part of their performance regalia. I will discuss the identity issue in more detail in chapter 7.

GOSPEL MUSIC AS PREFERRED GENRE

"Gospel music" as a religious music genre is hardly a bounded category. A distinction can be made between gospel songs, a genre heard in White evangelical denominations, and gospel as a Black American sacred music genre. The foundation for Black American gospel music rests in churches of the urban southern United States in the 1920s. Rooted in their African heritage and aesthetic ideals, Black gospel music integrates dance, handclapping, call-and-response singing, a percussive vocal technique, and the use of improvisation and the manipulation of pitch (Burnim 1985a). It has evolved into contemporary styles, characterized by the use of modern instruments that feature prominently in popular music genres, such as rhythm and blues, and soul; contemporary Black gospel shares common features of vocal techniques with these popular styles. As a sacred music genre, Black gospel music is a continuation of the creative expression of Black experiences, struggles, beliefs, values, and aesthetics, given theological interpretation in the context of modern circumstances (Burnim 2001).

In South Africa, two recognizable forms of singing are commonly called gospel music. The first is the gospel chorus (in Zulu, *amakhorasi*). *Amakhorasi* are short songs of usually one to two verses, plus a refrain. A gospel chorus is led by a soloist, who improvises on a few verses and may introduce several more in any given performance event by simply manipulating the theme and existing texts of the song while cueing the choir and congregation into the refrain, which is generally easy to memorize. The style is consistent with an African oral medium of performance, and the theme often speaks to individual and community experience, a personal relationship with God, repudiation of sin, rejection of Satan, salvation and peace with God, and eschatological vision. Lead soloists tend to reinforce these themes by inserting sermonettes and/or brief prayer formularies (discussed in details below). The style of singing is generally accompanied with handclapping and dance, and it resembles the indigenous form of vocal music.

In South Africa, the African independent churches were the earliest Christian groups to perform the *amakhorasi*—which explains its proximity to indigenous forms of vocal music. The advent of the American Pentecostal movements since the 1960s saw the popularization of this style of singing, but the mainstream denominations, such as the Roman Catholic, Anglican, Presbyterian, and Dutch Reformed churches, which had built the mission churches of the colonial era, frowned on the style of music until recently. Although they have now become more open to the performance of *amakhorasi* in their spaces, the style has yet to be fully integrated into their liturgical activities.

A second form of gospel music found its way onto the soundscape of South Africa again via the presence of Black American churches, including the African Methodist Episcopal Church and other evangelical groups. Mega churches modeled after those of the likes of Bishop T. D. Jakes[4] are now part of the urban culture, drawing in especially the younger generation of Black urban dwellers between the ages of 18 and 45. In Durban, the Durban Christian Center is a remarkable landmark. It holds up to two services every Sunday with approximately 7,000 youthful congregants. The congregation has grown mightily, prompting the erection of the Jesus Dome, a hall with a seating capacity of 5,000, which can be seen from the N-3 route on the way to Pinetown from Durban city. The music of these Pentecostal churches, like their Black American models, makes use of instruments of contemporary popular music, including drum sets, electric bass, synthesizers, electric guitars, and heavily amplified sound systems. Trained musicians often arrange the songs, though their arrangements are not often written down, but are performed by talented artists.

On another level, South Africa has seen streams of Black American gospel artists and their secular (especially soul) counterparts come and go, leaving their sonic imprints on the nation's soundscape. These artists have influenced numerous emergent gospel artists in South Africa. For example, Rebecca Malope, host of SABC's *Gospel Time*, celebrated in South Africa as the queen of South African gospel, discussed with the *Sunday Times* the formative years of her career as a gospel singer and the inspiration she drew from American soul singers: "I wanted to sing. I wanted to be like Donny Hathaway, Stevie Wonder, Anita Baker. But using my own voice" (*Sunday Times* 2008).

The emergent gospel artists of South Africa, including Rebecca Malope, Deborah Fraser, Sipho Makhabane, Mthunzi Namba, and Benjamin Dube, have successfully created a South African version of Black gospel by combining elements of Black American soul with their indigenous *amakhorasi* style. They articulate their individual experiences within the harsh economic, social, and political history of South Africa, and reformulate them as characteristic experiences of their communities and the society at large. Hence, they hold a perception of themselves as engaged in a ministry of bringing the gospel of hope to their audience and their people in the face of the social, economic, and political realities. It is in the light of this perceived sense of mission and ministry that one must appreciate Siphithemba's choice of gospel as its signature musical genre.

Members of Siphithemba made me understand that they preferred to be designated as a gospel choir, rather than as an HIV/AIDS choir. They saw themselves as engaged in the mission of preaching the gospel through their music and activities, which encapsulates the spirituality of hope and faith in God in the presence of HIV and AIDS. As to why they chose to perform gospel music and not other styles, such as hymns, Phumlani explained that they made a conscious choice to stick to gospel music, since there was a huge selection of songs that they could easily draw upon and that could easily relate to their experiences. In addition, they compose their own songs. Moreover, they were not trained in Western music, and so they have not had the ability to engage in extensive reading and interpretation of formally composed church hymns and other modern arrangements, even of those com posed by Africans.

The most commonly heard gospel tunes in South Africa, either on the radio waves or in churches, are those with simple repetitive refrains set to call-and-response patterns, but with room for elaborate solo improvisations. This style of music comprises the bulk of Siphithemba's repertoire. The songs are arranged, but not often written down. Xolani's response when I asked for the score of some of their songs, including those that they had adapted, was "you know *umfundisi,* these things, we just do them: it's difficult to see anybody who writes them down." Phumlani gave me a similar answer, but differentiated thus between gospel songs and formally composed art music that are used as set pieces for regional and national choral festivals:

> You know, I used to conductor my school choir during competitions. The songs for the competitions are like church hymns, or maybe sometimes the

> composers want to make them sound like classical music. Then you have to sing it that way, because the judges are looking at the song the way the composer wrote it. So if you sing it differently, you will fail. But this one [gospel songs], people can change it sometimes when they are singing it, because of the Holy Spirit.

Phumlani's statement points to characteristics of Black gospel music. The first is that, as elaborate as the gospel songs may be, they still belong in the African oral tradition. Second, Black gospel music, at least in South African contexts, has an elasticity that makes it adaptable to circumstances and experiences. As I show in this work, Siphithemba has successfully adapted preexisting gospel songs by giving them new interpretations in the light of their HIV/AIDS experience.

SIPHITHEMBA SONG THEMES

A conglomeration of themes in the choir's songs reveals its worldview regarding the HIV/AIDS struggle. The themes reveal Siphithemba's consciousness about dealing with HIV/AIDS as a form of battle, the collective effort required to wage the war against HIV/AIDS, and the emotional, spiritual, and physical attitudes that must accompany this fight. In this section, we see that Siphithemba members speak to themselves as much as they speak to their community. The themes in the songs form a dialogue with the audience about the reality of AIDS. Elements of history are invoked, meanings of original songs are transposed in new contexts and in the face of the new reality, and people are strengthened with the message of hope, even as they are challenged to change for good.

STRUGGLE AND MILITARISM

Former president Nelson Mandela in 1996 analyzed the HIV/AIDS pandemic in South Africa in light of apartheid and declared it the "next struggle" (Ndungane 2003:58). Since then, the act of linking HIV/AIDS with apartheid—even if only in symbolic ways—has become a major component of the AIDS discourse in South Africa. The annual world AIDS benefit pop music concert is named 46664 Concert, recalling Nelson Mandela's Robin Island prison number. Siphithemba appropriates this discourse by composing and performing songs that are imbued with a strong sense of urgency and militancy. At least five songs of Siphithemba's major repertoire have explicit references to arming and bearing arms: "Kulukhuni Ezweni" (It's Hard in this

World); "Izizwe Mazihlome" (The Nation Must Arm); "Ikhalaphi" (From Whence the Cry?); "Siyaphela Isizwe seNkosi" (The Nation of the Lord is Finishing), a reference to fighting and victory; and "Nkonyane Kandaba" (Son of Ndaba), originally a battlefield song.[5] Three are gospel songs, while two are preexisting Zulu traditional songs. Whereas the gospel songs mostly urge arming with knowledge as a weapon for the defeat of HIV/AIDS, the traditional songs, especially "Nkonyane Kandaba," have explicit reference to actual battlefield experience.

The song "Nkonyane Kandaba" illustrates the link between the current HIV/AIDS struggle and the antiapartheid struggle.[6]

Wathinta thina, wathinta abangasekufa,
Safa saphenduka, saphenduka injebomvu.
Solo: We Nkhonyane kandaba!
Chorus: Kwanyakaza umkhonto.
We nkonyane kandaba!

You've touched us, who die no more,
We die and we return [angry], like the red dog.
Solo: Oh you royal sons!
Chorus: The spears are moving.
Oh you royal sons!

The song depicts a people who have been wounded in battle, but who return stronger and braver, ready to engage the enemy once again, with even more determination to win. Two literary factors define the song however. One is the militarism of the text, exemplified in the reference to *umkhonto* 'spear,' the main war implement of Zulu infantry regiments. Important to the issue of the Zulu sense of militarism is the fact that they fight wars of self-defense. The opening line of the song makes explicit reference to acts of provocation, which must be responded to with ferocity. In other words, the Zulu nation and its people are portrayed as a peace-loving people. This is contrary to accounts in literature, which portrayed King Shaka and the Zulu as warmongers, a pugnacious tribal entity (Wylie 2006). This manner of responding to provocation is not lost in history. When the performance of *ngoma* dance emerged as part of Black urban form of resistance to White domination in the first quarter of the twentieth century, the tone of the songs continued to underscore the fact that they had been provoked and their rights violated. An example is found in the lines of the defiant song performed by the ICU *ngoma* dancers in Durban, on one January night in 1930. An Englishwoman Alison Wessels, to whom George Champion, leader of the ICU, provided the meaning, documented a song thus (see Perham 1974: 196),

Who has taken our country from us?
[. . .] The land was ours; now it is taken
[. . .] Come out and fight!
[. . .] Shame on the man who is burnt in his hut!

The other factor is the reference to Ndaba, Shaka's great-grandfather, which has a nationalist underpinning, whereby *Konyane Kandaba* 'young one of Ndaba'[7] simply refers to the Zulu. As an industrializing urban Black culture, a pervasive sense of nationalism characterized the performance of Zulu vocal music.

It is unclear how old the song is and who its original composer was, but it gained popularity through Mbogeni Ngema's musical *Sarafina*, which was later turned into a movie. First performed as a musical at the Market Theatre in Johannesburg in June 1987, *Sarafina* depicts the Soweto students' uprising in 1976. In 1992, it was adapted into a movie featuring Hollywood star Whoopi Goldberg, with Leleti Khumalo as Sarafina (*Sarafina* [1987] 2002).

In the musical *Sarafina*, Mbogeni Ngema inserted the song immediately following the scene where Sabela, the Black constable, beats and kicks Koku under the supervision of two White officers, as he transverses the neighborhoods of Soweto to meet Sarafina. The White officers then set the dog on Koku, which bites him deep in the leg as he tries to jump the fence. The act of brutality meted out on Koku prompts the students to declare war on the apartheid police and resolve to fight the system. In a similar way, Siphithemba members show a clear consciousness about their experience of HIV/AIDS as a struggle, but also they construe it as a struggle for their community. By invoking the name of Ndaba in the song, they symbolically link their present experience with wars the Zulu have fought and won, or at least survived. After all, they are the descendants of Ndaba, the great-grandfather of Shaka, the brave leader and army commander, and founder of the great kingdom. They have had many struggles, and have passed through and survived several ordeals. Hence, they believe not only that they can defeat the virus, but that their community can emerge stronger and better as a result.

FAITH AND HOPE

The name *Siphithemba* (We Give Hope) speaks volumes about the faith and hope that the choir and its members bear. This sentiment was nurtured at the Sinkithemba AIDS clinic of McCord Hospital. For the Siphithemba Choir, faith and trust in God is the foundation of their struggle with the virus. In their music, faith and hope are reflected in different ways. Sometimes a seeming sense of despair, as in "Kulukhuni Ezweni" (It's Hard in This World) gives rise to a sudden surge in hope and trust in what God is about to do.

Kulukhuni Ezweni (*It's Hard in this World) By Phumlani*

Kulukhuni 'madoda,
Kulukhuni ezweni,
Kulukhuni 'madoda
Oh kulukhuni.

Kutheni na?
Kutheni na,
Thixo Somandla?

We maZulu hlomani,
We maZulu hlomani,
Hayi hayi, we maZulu hlomani.

Siyahamba madoda,
Siyahamba siy'ekhaya ezulwini.
Kumnandi kunokuthula,
Hayi kunokuthula.

Ekhaya lakho Baba,
Ekhaya lakho Baba akufiwa.
Ngifisa' ukuwubona,
Lombuso wezulu lakho.

It's hard men,
It's hard in this world.
It's hard men oh!
Oh it's hard.

What is it?
What is it,
Father God?

Zulu be armed,
Zulu be armed,
hayi hayi Zulu be armed.

We're going men,
We're going home to heaven.

It's nice and peaceful,
Hayi it is peaceful.

At your home, Father,
At your home, Father, there is no death.
I wish to see (it),
Your heavenly kingdom.

The hope that is mixed with the seeming sense of despair often comes out being teleological and eschatological—looking beyond the here and now to the ultimate peace and tranquility of God's kingdom. Other examples of such themes are found in songs such as "Ngizohamba" (I'm Going), which was adapted by Phumlani, the choir conductor:

Ngizohamba, ngiyekhaya,
Ngiyolungisa indawo,
Ngoba ekhaya likaBaba,
Kunezindlu eziningi.
I'm going, I'm going home,
I'll be okay in that place,
Because at [my] Father's house,
There are many houses[8]

Rhythm change with dance
Call/Response: Maningakhathazeki,
Kholwani uBaba.
Izinhliziyo zenu mazingakhathazeki.
Izinhliziyo zenu zingakkathazeki.

Call/Response: Do not worry,
Believe in (my) Father.
Your hearts should not worry.
Your hearts should not worry.

Or still in Phakamile's "Praises":
We [shall] sing praises.
We praise you Lord,
'Cause we know that resurrection day
Is coming soon.
We better hold on,
Hold on,
'Cause we know that resurrection day
Is coming soon.

The eschatological vision therefore mitigates the feeling of despair, and thereby informs the reason to sing songs like "In Times of Sorrow":
Lord, I love you.
Lord, I need you.
Lord, I trust you.
Lord, I praise you,
In times of sorrows and happiness.

Ngiyakuthanda.
Ngiyakudinga.
Nguyakwethemba,
Njalo njalo,
Ebuhleni nasebubini.

I love you.
I need you.
I trust in you,
Always, always,
In good and in bad times.

Call: In moments like this,
Choral response: I sing aloud the song;
I sing aloud the song unto Jesus.
Call: In moments like this,
Response: I sing aloud the song;
I sing aloud the song unto Him.
Call: Singing,
Response: I love you, Lord;
I love you, Lord; I love you, Lord.

After the last phrase, the choir hums. Faith in God and consciousness about what God is doing for them creates upbeat moments in songs such as in "Yes, My Lord," composed by Phumlani:

Leader: Yes, my Lord,
Choir: Yes, yes, yes.
Yes, my Lord. (2x)
Leader: We ought to praise you, Lord,
Choir: Oh yeah!
(repeat)

Leader: Jump, jump, jump, jump!
Choir: Yes, yes, yes, yes, my Lord.

We ought to praise you, Lord,
Oh yeah!
(repeat)

Dance, dance, dance, dance!
Choir: Yes, yes, yes, yes, my Lord.

Leader: We ought to praise you, Lord,
Choir: Oh yeah!

Leader: *Siguqa ngamadolo* ['Let's kneel down', as choir kneels]
Choir: Yes, yes, yes, yes, my Lord. (2x)

The messages in these songs are not meant for the singers alone: they are also meant to bring hope to their audience. The HIV/AIDS pandemic has created an unprecedented degree of depression, especially in the South African Black community, second only to that experienced under apartheid, and sometimes worse. It is hard to see any family or individual person who has not been affected by AIDS directly or indirectly. Thus the choir sings their faith and hope, and brings it to share with their audience and community, who must live by faith and hope in God as the ultimate answer to the problem.

ON BEHAVIOR CHANGE

The need for behavior change as a major preventive tool against the spread of HIV/AIDS is a dominant theme in the current HIV/AIDS discourse. In 2007, the Gauteng Provincial Government rolled out a preventive program that was rallying more than 12,000 volunteers, who distributed leaflets door to door and talked to people about the need for changing social behaviors that exposed them to the risk of HIV/AIDS. The leaflets had persuasive messages from religious leaders, musicians, and judges, calling on young people to "delay their sex debut," and for married couples to remain faithful in their relationships, or at least to embrace "condomization." This practice was replicated in other provinces such as KwaZulu-Natal, coupled with the use of multiple other media platforms to disseminate messages of disease prevention. The call for "delay[ed] sex debut" is still the same in the story of the awarding of university scholarship to sixteen female students in the Uthukela District of KwaZulu-Natal which I referenced earlier in chapter 4.

For the members of Siphithemba, however, preventive measures begin with knowledge of one's status. Their conviction that preventive measures begin with knowledge of one's status is borne out in members' crusade in their communities, in which they encourage people to be tested. Phumlani,

Zinhle, Phakamile, and Nomusa all testify to having successfully persuaded their family members and friends to be tested and get appropriate help.

The case of South Africa is exacerbated by poverty inherited from decades of apartheid and economic marginalization of Africans and its accompanying migrant labor system (Meadows 2003: 154). In my experience of living in South Africa while conducting this research, I saw that the migrant labor system has not yet vanished completely amid the progress that the ANC-led government has made in human and economic development. Even in the Catholic Pastoral Center where I lived, most of the Black male and female service staff lived in single rooms in the center without their partners and children. They did not have enough time during the month to travel to the rural areas to visit their families, so they remained in the center during their 1½ to 2 off-days every fortnight.

It is not only the migrant workers who are exposed to the dangers of indulging in behaviors inimical to their health, but even the wives, husbands, and teenage children they leave at home. Two sample traditional songs by the choir- "isiyalo" (advice) and "ikhalaphi" (from whence the cry) speak eloquently to the issue of the loss of traditional values and moral rectitude. The two songs speak about promiscuous lifestyles, touching on the theme of sexuality integral to HIV/AIDS discourse. The choir uses these two songs as means of engaging in the conversations on disease prevention through behavioral change.

Set in a classic call-and-response pattern, and often performed to the accompaniment of a recorded background track paired with a choreographed form of Zulu *ngoma* dance, isiyalo speaks about a young beautiful lady who engages in prostitution while rejecting the men who propose marriage to her.

Isiyalo

Call: Asikho isiyalo la izalwakhona,
Resp: Asikh' isiyalo la izalwakhona.
Iphum' ekhaya igqoke kahle,
Ifike ngalena kwendaba,
Ekumule idilozi ilibeke phansi,
Thubhobho i-gemu.
Asikh' isiyalo la izalwakhona.

Refrain (with solo improvisation)
Call: Ayivumi ngishela kwaMasondo ayivumi,
Resp: Ngishela kwaMasondo ayivumi.
Call: Le'ntombi yenzani?
Resp: Ngishela kwaMansondo ayivumi.

Call: There's no advice from whence she comes,
Resp: There's no advice from whence she comes.
She comes from home well dressed,
She comes across the hill,
She strips pants and puts it down,
For a 20 cents game.
There's no advice from whence she comes.

Refrain (with solo improvisation)
Call: She rejects my proposal to kwaMasondo,
Resp: I propose [to] kwaMasondo, she refuses.
Call: What is the young lady doing?
Resp: I propose [to] kwaMasondo, she refuses.

Isiyalo depicts a "beautiful one" (KwaMasondo)[9] with no parental guidance, resulting in her reckless sexual lifestyle. The refrain part of the song highlights KwaMasondo's rejection of marriage and her preference for prostitution.

Ikhalaphi, on the other hand, speaks about a female lover whose sagging breasts are clear indications that she is engaging in pre-marital sex.

Ikhalaphi

A

Call: Ikhalaphi (con locutae)?
Resp: Ikhalaphi induku yempi?
Sizwa ngosi, ikhalaphi.

B

Call: Awe kanjani?
Resp: Awe knajani?
Amabele ejongosi,
Okusho ukuthi seliphuma kanje
Call: Wetshitshi lami!
Call: Awusho ngani?
Resp: Uma usuphuma kanje?
Call: Awusho ngani?
Resp: Awusho, uma usuphuma kanje?
Call: Ikhalaphi (con locutae)?
Resp: Ikhalaphi induku yempi?
Sizwa ngosi, ikhalaphi.

B

Call: How did they (breasts) fall?
Resp: How did they fall?

The breasts of the virgin,
It means that she is (already) having affairs.
Call: Oh my virgin (girl)!
Call: Why did you not tell me?
Resp: When you started affairs?
Call: Why did you not tell me?
Resp: Why not, when you started affairs?

On another level, the two songs, especially "isiyalo" connects with the story of migrant labor system that has persisted, albeit in a new way, in post-apartheid South Africa, and which has been noted to contribute to the spread of HIV/AIDS. The dismantling of apartheid following the ushering in of majority democratic rule in 1994 precipitated a massive population influx into urban areas from rural communities in the hope of making a better living. Unfortunately dangerous lifestyles often become the characteristic consequence of the failed dreams, resulting thus in large numbers of migrant sex workers, whose urban clients are domestic workers, service laborers, and tourists (Hunter 2007: 689–700).

I pointed it out to the choir members that the songs appear to focuses exclusively on the sexual behavior of girls, and not on that of the men. It may reinforce the problems of gender disparity that are witnessed in the HIV/AIDS and STI discourse, which often works against women. But Wicky and Nomusa, female members of the choir, did not appear to have problem with the representation. According to Wicky, "The song is saying the right thing, because that is actually what is happening." Nomusa insisted that there is no need to worry about the gender representation, since the songs are still true and relevant in the light of present-day social realities:

> Well that is something that does happen. You'll find a girl leaving home in a good-looking manner; then they reach a certain place; then they have to change. The song doesn't just talk about the clothing: it talks about something that they end up doing. . . . Because it is something that happens. We know that it happens, so it doesn't bother us that much.

The fact still remains that no female prostitute is successful in her business without male clients. The economic gains made in South Africa since 2000 have seen many young Black men become economically buoyant via the government policy of Black economic empowerment. Many men are now living extravagant lifestyles, with a mix of some degree of irresponsibility, evidenced in the cars they drive and the girlfriends they have. Based on the knowledge that I gained by interacting daily with some university students who resided at the Glenmore Pastoral Center, among female college students, a new language has emerged as a way of referencing their male patrons and "sugar daddies" as they engage in transactional sex. Some girls have a minister of education (one who pays for their education), a minister of transport (one who provides them transport fare), a minister of housing (one who pays for their accommodation), and a minister of communications (one who buys them cell phones and supplies them airtime). Thus, it is clear, men and women alike are involved in the "20-cent game."

STIGMA AND DENIAL

The issue of behavior change is linked to denial. Denial manifests itself at individual and public levels of policymaking. The denial that I am concerned mostly with here, and as far as Siphithemba's music is concerned, is that at the individual level. Siphithemba members all agree that denial stems from ignorance of one's status, and what I call a pathological entrenchment in the myths about HIV/AIDS, which in turn fuels the stigma system that mitigates the containment of the virus. The choir's call for people to know their status is therefore also a call against living in denial of the reality of the disease.

Unfortunately, testing in South African is often thought to reveal positive status, and the fact that testing also identifies those who are negative is frequently ignored. Several young people in the course of this research admitted that they were full of anxiety about their status, and were thus afraid to be tested. The danger inherent in this reticence is perpetual anxiety—stress, depression, and despair, particularly with persons who may have lost intimate partners and close relatives to the virus. For this reason, the use of the biblical verse "You shall know the truth, and the truth shall make you free" (John 8:32) has become a mainstay in the HIV/AIDS denial discourse in church quarters. The Rev. Mandla Mdabe, an HIV-positive Methodist minister, drums it in hard during most of his motivational talks at HIV/AIDS workshops, such as the one at St. Clement Home-Based Care Project AIDS Awareness Function in 2007 and during a workshop at the Diakonia Center in Durban in 2012. The Cape Town Anglican Archbishop Ndungane fears that "to accept less than knowing [our status and] our partner's status is to risk our suicide" (2003: 61). Although Siphithemba has no song that incorporates this biblical verse, other groups have produced songs that speak strongly about stress resulting from refusal to know one's status. A theater group from Clermont, also based at the St. Clement Catholic Church, incorporates songs and dances in its theater productions designed for HIV/AIDS education. One of its songs makes explicit use of this biblical verse:

The truth shall set you free.
Know your HIV status now.
Be free from stress; go for blood test,
So that you could know your status.

On another level, denial in South Africa is fueled by a common attitude of men who tend to believe that HIV is women's problem, and by the myth that links HIV/AIDS to witchcraft. During the course of this research, I visited several HIV/AIDS support groups in the Ethekwini District. I observed that most of these groups were composed exclusively of women. In each instance, I sought to understand the reason for the absence of men, and the women always responded: "Our men are stubborn; they live in denial." Yet many of these women live with spouses and boyfriends, many of whom may actually be infected, but refuse to be tested, even after they have become sick.

Denial resulting from attributing HIV/AIDS to witchcraft is exemplified in an experience I had while embarking on a home visitation with the St. Clement Catholic Home-Based Care Project in May of 2007. We had left the center at about 9:00 a.m. one day to visit sick patients at the KwaDabeka section of Clermont. Usually home visitations lasted until about 1:00 p.m., when we would return to pick up food and go for dishing. But on this day, at 11:00 a.m., Ugogo[10] called us to return immediately and pick up a sick patient to be dropped off at the township's polyclinic. The patient was a woman with two children, both of whom were under five years of age. The woman confirmed that she had AIDS, and evidently she was sick with anemia, had lost a lot of weight, and was unable to walk on her own. She was simply bedridden. Her boyfriend was a young man in his mid-thirties to early forties. Although he still looked somewhat healthy and strong, he had a rash on his body and appeared to be losing weight. Given the situation, the nursing sister that was with us suggested that he see a counselor with the kids while the girlfriend was being monitored. She suggested further that he should consider having the children tested for HIV. But the young man insisted that he and his children were all healthy and did not have HIV/AIDS. According to him, his girlfriend's sickness was a result of *umuthi*[11] being sent upon them by their neighbors' witchcraft activities. This form of denial is a major factor in exacerbating the spread of the disease. Unfortunately, the discourse on denial in South Africa has focused on the government and its policies (Nattrass 2007), and less on the individual and behavior that requires change.

From their own experiences, Siphithemba members understand the dangers inherent in denial of all sorts. Some women in the group tell personal stories about how upon learning about their HIV-positive status through prenatal testing, they were deserted by their male partners, who denied having anything to do with their being infected. These men often ended up with other women and thereby exposed more people to the risk of being infected. It explains why many of the choir members have embarked on persuading family members and relatives—and often successfully—to know their status by testing.

As far as denial comes out of ignorance—that of refusal to know one's status, as well as ignorance arising from myths about HIV/AIDS—so it breeds forms of stigma that are built on ignorance. Two types of stigma are particularly important to discuss here: namely, that people living with AIDS are positive because they are sinners; and that people living with AIDS are so weak and moribund that they cannot live productive lives.

The first stigma arises from the myth that HIV/AIDS is a curse from God as punishment for the sins of people as has been propagated by some evangelical preachers such as Billi Graham and Jerry Falwell (Kopelman 2002; Chikwem et al., 2003: 1). Simialrly, Roger Cardinal Mahony, former Archbishop of Los Angeles, who shortly after returning from the enclave that elected Pope Benedict XVI responded to questions on CNN about what the new pope would do about AIDS in Africa. He remarked that the problem of HIV/AIDS in Africa is simply that of promiscuity. The remarks by religious leaders thus make the church most guilty of stigmatization, despite all its good work. For in these remarks, those who are HIV-positive have had to bear the extra burden of being looked upon as victims of their own immorality. The type of comment from a prince of the Roman Catholic Church is part of what fuels the endless battle against stigmatizing people living with AIDS. As Archbishop Ndungane has rightly observed, "the Church plays a critical role in shaping the values *and attitudes* of a community *towards the HIV/AIDS victims*" (2003: 61, italics added).

Several reports coming out from world institutions like the UN, WHO, UNICEF, USAIDS, and from church institutions at national and international levels, such as the World Council of Churches and the Diakonia Council of Churches, identify the economic, political, social, and environmental conditions that fuel the spread of HIV and AIDS.[12] While it still remains true that "sexual behaviors of people must change in order to save lives" (Ndungane 2003: 60), greater progress could be made by working to improve people's living conditions. The HIV virus is not a sin, says Archbishop Ndugane, and any continued attempt to moralize the disease confuses people all the more, and minimizes the successes that could be scored in the current struggle. Moreover, when victims of the human immunodeficiency virus are looked upon as immoral, they become double victims in the circumstances of the same disease.

Finally, looking at people living with AIDS as coffin-bound largely results from the pictures of bedridden, terminally ill patients that the media—particularly Western media, reporting on Africa—projects to their audience.[13] Siphithemba members have defied this picture by adopting a positive lifestyle. For them positive living means taking their treatment seriously, being economically self-reliant, and engaging in industry. Touring North America and Europe has helped them dispel the fears that people have of them as imminently terminal, or as unproductive. In fact, it has even earned them envy and jealousy from people who have moralistic attitudes toward them. It was in response to this attitude that Sizwe Ndlela composed the song "Sizwile Ukuthi" (We Heard the Gossip- to be analyzed in detail in chapter 6), which shows the extent to which Siphithemba would go to fight against being stigmatized, and proves that people are their own best advocates against the burden of stigma.

SUMMARY AND CONCLUSION

In conclusion, my aim in this chapter has been to describe, in as much detail as possible, the preferred genres and thematic content of Siphithemba songs and how these articulate with the choir members' experience of HIV/AIDS, which forms part of the larger societal experience of the disease. Hence, they are deeply engaged in ongoing conversations about HIV/AIDS, both within South Africa and abroad. The politics, myths, social epidemiology, and economy of HIV/AIDS are not lost to them: instead, these issues come to bear on the kind of music they make, and the themes they address in their songs.

I submit that the Siphithemba choir not only sings about HIV/AIDS, but actually performs HIV/AIDS as human experience—of the member themselves, their local community, South Africa, and the world. They bring their African worldview to the fore, making the context of their musical performance an arena where competing ideas play out, and at the same time are reconciled as integral factors to deal with their struggle. In the end, hope—and hope alone—stands out as the guiding principle in their entire endeavor.

NOTES

1. http://dogreatthings.co.za/music/2015-prescribed-music/ (accessed February 14, 2016).

2. For more details on this concept, see Germond and Molapo (2006).

3. The two songs are from Hugh Tracey's collection, courtesy of ILAM, Rhodes University, Grahamstown South Africa.

4. T. D. Jakes is the pastor of The Potter's House, a 30,000 member nondenominational mega church in Dallas, Texas. He is reckoned as "the premiere contemporary spiritual voice" in North America, particularly in the African American community. With a special interest in the continent of Africa, his FAITH FOR AFRICA initiative is active in east and southern Africa (see "Biography," http://www.tdjakes.com/site/PageServer?pagename=about_biography, accessed on 10 August 2009).

5. Nkonyane KaNdaba is the praise name for the Zulu chiefdom under the Mthetwa confederacy. It was derived from Ndaba, the great-grandfather of Shaka, who is the progenitor of the Zulu chiefdom. In the pre-Shaka Zulu nation, military regiments were organized according to chiefdoms, but perhaps for security reasons against treason, Shaka changed the formations into age-grade regiments. In this battle

song, the sons of the chiefdom are urged to proceed into battle with the ferocity of wounded dogs.

6. The song, according to Xolani Zulu, was associated mostly with the Umkhonto Wesizwe (Spear of the Nation), the military wing of the African National Congress. It became more popular after Mbogeni Ngema adapted it in his movie-turned-musical *Sarafina* at the Johannesburg Market Theatre in 1987.

7. *Nkonyane* in Zulu is a 'young horse,' but it has the transferred sense of 'youthful man.'

8. This is a reference to John 14:2, a biblical passage in which Jesus is asserting his identity with the Father, and that belief in him equals belief in the Father. Hence the response "Believe in (my) Father."

9. 'KwaMasondo' is Zulu referent for a beautiful one.

10. *Ugogo* means 'grandmother,' but Mrs. Mlambo, the mother of South Africa's former deputy president Phumzile Mlabmbo-Ngcuka and coordinator of the St. Clement Home-Based Care Project, was called by this name by everyone who worked at the Home-Based Care Project.

11. *Umuthi* in Zulu means 'traditional medicine, charm,' usually used to cure ailments, to protect against spiritual attacks, or still to inflict spiritual harm on a person that would manifest in the form of physical ailment. The charm is often performed in a witchcraft system known in Zulu as *Ubuthakathi.*

12. See, for example, the *Oikos Journey* (2006).

13. For more on the media images, see Okigbo and Ezumah (2015), "Media Health Images of Africa and the Politics of Representation." *Journal of Asian and African Studies.*

Chapter 6

Creative Processes and Musical Stylistics

Individual members of the choir have composed most of the Siphithemba's repertoire, but they draw from a large repository of gospel and traditional music, which they reworked by way of adaptation or quotation to fit their experience of HIV and AIDS, and to transmit messages to local audiences in recognizable forms. Their artistic techniques exhibit their ingenuity in drawing upon and transforming their immediate soundscape to speak to themselves and their community. In this chapter, I devote attention to the creative process by which the choir generates its repertoire and the stylistics of its musical performances.

Although individual members are encouraged to compose songs according to personal inspirations, some of their most effective songs are those that they created through collaborative effort, what I call communal approach to composition. I suggest that this approach is in fact indexical of the Zulu sense of *ubuntu*, which permeates their activities and organization. I also examine their performance practice and how their styles and techniques of delivery help to frame the meanings and messages they seek to convey in any given music event. To do this, I will inevitably revisit some songs that have already been analyzed in the previous chapters of this work. My focus however is the process by which the individual songs were created, and how the choir has performed them, without reintroducing analyses that had already been done.

COMMUNAL COMPOSITIONAL PRACTICE

The process of song composition in the Siphithemba Choir is an example of communal action in which individuals have an opportunity to express their experiences in music and merge them with those of other members.

Many songs are composed by individual members, including especially those by Phumlani, Sizwe, and Phakamile. A mixture of melancholy and hope often characterizes the songs, yet they speak to the experiences and imaginations of all. An example is "Kulukhuni Ezweni" (It's Hard in This World), composed by Phumlani (see song text in chapter 4). The song is a soliloquy seeking to engage in conversation with: (1) those who share the experience of being HIV-positive and (2) God, to question the reason for the scourge of the disease. The text rallies his compatriots to rise up and fight, signaling a sudden outburst of energy and resilience, and then ending with hope and vision of spiritual triumph over these earthly ordeals in the heavenly kingdom. One sees in the song a paradox of relationship between temporal and spiritual orders: the former full of ordeals, and the later an escape from the temporal. Ncamisile and Sizile, two members of the choir, resolved the paradox for me one Sunday evening as we drove from Umlazi to the city, to drop Sizile off at the Inanda taxi station. I raised the question about how they can sing about the world as full of ordeals that must be escaped to the bliss of heaven while asking the Zulu to rise up, arm, and fight it. Sizile answered "*Umfundisi*, what are we supposed to do? We cannot just give up because of what happened to us." Ncamisile added, "It is also how we feel about the whole thing. For me sometimes, I think I should die and forget everything. But I also know that I will die when God wants me. I can still do something now that I am alive."

Ncamisile's and Sizile's explanation resonated with Phumlani's explanation about positive living, which Phumlani explained as embracing the situation and encouraging oneself and others to be proactive in improving their lives despite being HIV-positive. Hence the insertion of the willingness and determination to engage in a struggle that must transform this temporal order into a state and place of survival, peace, and tranquility, which prefigures that which is anticipated in the bliss of God's abode. This contemplative experience is not unique to Phumlani: it is one with which other Siphithemba members easily identify.

The analysis above speaks of individual compositions which, speak to the experience of the choir members, but much of Siphithemba's repertoire is group-composed. Information gathered from Phumlani and Xolani, and observation of the choir at rehearsals, show that communal composition occurs in three ways: (1) choir members adapt, rearrange, and insert a message into preexisting song tunes, to, according to Xolani "connect with what they already know;" (2) choir members contribute bits of and pieces of ideas which are then assembled and synthesized into one and then set to music, or (3) a new theme and textual message is hammered into a melody that has been created and harmonized by the group through humming. These themes are often created out of individual experiences and issues that affect their community. Anybody present is free to add to this message until a fully composed song emerges. Another avenue the group takes is to identify a theme and invite everybody to compose something about it, based on personal and community experience. The choir members integrate all the contributions into one, and then they seek to turn the text into song.

One song that illustrates this communal approach to composition in process as in lyrical content and performance is "Siyaphela IsiZwe seNkosi" (The nation of the Lord is finishing) (see appendix for notational transcription).

Siyaphela

A

a.

Siyaphela isizwe seNkosi
Sibulawa ngumashayabhuqe
Vukani maAfrika silwenawo
The nation of the Lord is finishing
Because its being killed by AIDS
Wake up Africa and fight with it

b.

If you are infected
We are also affected
Come on Africa
Let's stand up and fight
Together we stand
But divided we fall
[*Transition with brief instrumental interlude*]

B

Refrain
Call: Yaze yankulu lendaba
Resp: Yaze yankulu lendaba
Call: Sizomnqoba?
Resp: Sizomnqoba kanjani lomashaya bhuqe?
Ulwazi loyamnqoba umashaya bhuqe
Call: Imishanguzo
Resp: Imishanguzo iyamthiba umashaya bhuqe
Ijazi liyamvimba umishaya bhuqc
Call: Ithemba
Resp: Ithemba liyaphilisa kulomashaya bhuqe
[This is a big issue
Resp: This is a big issue

Call: Shall we conquer it?
Resp: How shall we conquer this AIDS?
Knowledge can conquer AIDS
Call: ARV
Resp: ARVs can prevent the spread of AIDS
Condoms can prevent the spread of AIDS
Call: Hope
Resp: Hope gives life with this AIDS]

C

[*Choreographed Dance Movement and instrumental break then a return to* B]

"Siyaphela Isizwe seNkosi" is set in homophonic A and rudimentary call-response B sections separated by a two-measure instrumental break, followed by a long dance and instruments break or C section. The A section has smaller internal segments of a and b that are repeated each. Hence the form of the song may be represented thus ||A a:||b:|| B || C||.

The choir generally attributes the composition of "Siyaphela" to Phumlani and Sizwe, although according to Phumlani, when they brought the song to the group, other members contributed to the final version. From Phumlani's account, the a segment of the first section came largely from Sizwe's inspiration, and the b segment was Phumlani's. They had agreed to write a song that spoke to their experience of the HIV/AIDS in their local community, and what must be done to curb its onslaught. This was the central message, and they began by writing the lyrics. It does not seem that a conscious decision was made about the language of the song, but when the English b segment of section A appeared to blend well with the message of the a segment, the decision was made to juxtapose them in the same section as it is now. Other choir members' input was mainly in the B section, where various ideas about how to conquer the disease are declared. These ideas are not new (in fact, they comprise part of the watchword in the general AIDS discourse in South Africa), but the idea of hope, as a source of life in the presence of the AIDS problem, is uniquely a Siphithemba signature slogan. Also, the choir members suggested the Zulu words that best describe the concept of AIDS (*umashaya bhuqe*), condom (*ijazi*), and antiretrovirals (*imishanguzo*) drawing from some of the slogans that are circulating in the public domain and turning them into nomenclatures in their songs. Finally, largely Sizwe, with the help of Phumlani, made the musical arrangement.

The a and b internal segments of the A section are differentiated only by lyrical content and language (IsiZulu and English respectively), but unified by melodic commonality. Also, the a segment ends in a half cadence, leaving a feeling of suspense, which calls for resolution. The yearning created by the suspense is immediately filled with the quick introduction of the b segment, which again quickly leaves the audience with a feeling of more suspense, by ending once again in a half cadence. The suspense, however, is immediately subsumed in the vocal gestures, such as ululations and the instrumental beats, which form the interlude with the instrumental and give a sense that something new is about to happen.

The two segments are set to three-part homophonic harmonic structure with mostly parallel thirds and sixths in triadic progression. This style of harmonic progression, is characteristic of Black South African adaptations of European hymn singing and their effort to harmonize the melodies. Many earlier researchers on Black choral singing observed the omnipresence of the parallel thirds and sixths in triadic harmonies. Speight, for instance, wrote "the natives are natural harmonizers. On hearing a melody played over, they will, without premeditation, drop into part-singing. They are especially fond of thirds and sixths, which they like to render with full sonority" (1934: 352).

South African musicologist David Dargie described this style of harmony as "Afro-diatonic harmony," and he suggested that it is a parallel triad-chord system that developed out of Africans' adaptation of the Western diatonic system of scale and harmony, as in the white keys of the piano. This style of harmonization is guided by the ear, wherein, everyone sings in a part with which he or she is comfortable, often moving in parallel with the melody (Dargie 1997:320). The aurality of the style of harmony is evidenced in the fact that Siphithemba's songs are all learned by rote, and are never written down. Sometimes the choristers tended to sound discordant notes as they endeavored to harmonize the melodies of their songs from their assigned vocal parts. In several rehearsal sessions, Sizwe would sit on the keyboard and remind the various parts what their lines ought to sound like. Even during the learning of new songs, he would allow the voices to attempt to harmonize the melody as it was laid out, then he would come back to fix the discordant spots. The homophonic harmonic structure is indicative of the hymnodic declamatory style, with its didactic outlook. The choir thus continues to maintain its European missionary musical heritage, meshed with its African musical techniques and aesthetic ideals.

The instrumental break between segments a and b in section A is two measures, with vocal gestures that signal that something is about to happen. The gestures include sounds like *hamba* 'go on' or 'proceed,' *yebo* 'yes, it is so,' and *haibo,* a gesture of surprise, usually accompanied with the raising of the eyebrows. The Zulu generally use such gestures to encourage a person's or group's actions. The gestures are acclamations and affirmations in and of themselves. In a Siphithemba performance event, members use them to acknowledge, acclaim, and affirm individual lead soloists or dancers when they are about to move to the front of the stage to lead the song, or to demonstrate a dance. In this particular music, they use the gestures to acknowledge and acclaim the soloist, who moves to the front of the group to lead the call-and-response B section.

The B section is actually set like a solo with a choral obbligato. Usually performed by Sizile, or in her absence another female member of the choir, the soloist is free to add texts to her part, including vocative sounds, like *eh!, oh!* or sometimes even words such as *mama* 'mother.' She could manipulate her pitch and vocal timbre, extend the vocative sounds through several measures at will, and use a disjunctive melodic flourish, which sometimes covers up to three octaves. In some performances, Phumlani adds to Sizile's part by layering his male solo vocal part over hers, but usually without letting her voice be drowned out.

Fundamentally, the solo part introduces the ideas that are heard in the choral response. In the first idea, she declares that *this is a big issue,* and the choir responds with her exact texts. In the subsequent ideas, she calls out only the first words, and the choir takes up their parts set to full statements. Although the choral responses to the solo calls are set, they lean completely on the soloists with respect to how many times each idea is to be declared. Thus, the length of the B section is not standard, compared with the A section. It could get longer or shorter in any given performance, depending on how many times the soloist chooses to repeat ideas that are being declared. The implication is that when the choir performs to the prerecorded sound track, the return to B after the choreographed dance and instrumental break could be so short sometimes that only the first idea is reintroduced, and the rest is cut off as soon as the recording fades out.

This process of musical composition and performance that I have discussed hereby reiterates what scholars have often noted about communal composition strategies in African (and African American) music (Burnim 2006:59; Henderson 1995:136) and musical performance (Nketia 1974:21–34; Stone 2005: 64–67). The communality of the compositional process shows that individual experience and effort must engage the struggle, but that they are most effective when they are joined with those of other members of the community.

Musical Adaptation

The practice of adapting preexisting gospel songs follows the process of individual and collective effort. This process can entail melodic and formal alteration of songs, but most especially it involves textual alteration, in which new texts related to the experience of the community replace the original ones. An example of such a song is "Izizwe Mazihlome" (The Nation Must Arm), adapted by Phumlani, Sizwe, and Xolani.

A. Nguyelo uJeso (or Usomandla),
Owayekhona ekuqaleni,
namhlanje.
Kuze nguye namhlanje

B. Call: Izizwe mazihlome bo,
Resp: Izizwe azihlome nasi isifo sihlasele.
Call: Izizwe mazihlome bo,
Res: Izizwe azihlome nalubhubhane luhlasele.
Call: Izizwe mazihlome bo,
Resp: Izizwe azihlome naligciwane lihlasele.
Call: Zingahlomi ngezibhamu,
Res: Zihlome ngolwazi lokuvikele ubhubhane.

C. Soli: Abstain!
Choir: Zihlome ngolwazi lokuvikele ubhubhane.
Soli: Be faithful!
Choir: Zihlome ngolwazi lokuvikele ubhubhane.
Soli: Condomize!
Choir: Zihlome ngolwazi lokuvikele ubhubhane.
Soli: Vaccine!
Choir: Zihlome ngolwazi lokuvikele ubhubhane.
C[1]Soli S/A: Uma ufakijazi uzosinda.
Choir: Zihlome ngolwazi lokuvikele ubhubhane
S/A Call: Uma ufakijazi uzophepha.
Choir: Zihlome ngolwazi lokuvikele ubhubhane.

Recapitulation
B. Call: Izizwe mazihlome bo,
Resp: Izizwe azihlome nasi isifo sihlasele.
Call: Izizwe mazihlome bo,
Resp: Izizwe azihlome nalubhubhane luhlasele.
Resp: Izizwe azihlome naligciwane lihlasele.
Call: Zingahlomi ngezibhamu,
Resp: Zihlome ngolwazi lokuvikele ubhubhane.

A. This is Jesus,
Who was there in the beginning,
He is still here even now.

B. Call: The nation must arm,
Resp: The nation must arm for the disease that is attacking us.
Call: The nation must arm,

Resp: The nation must arm for the disease that is attacking us.
Call: The nation must arm,
Resp: The nation must arm for the disease that is attacking us.
Call: They mustn't arm with guns,
Resp: But with knowledge of disease prevention.

C. Soli: Abstain!
Choir: Arm with knowledge of disease prevention.
Soli: Be faithful!
Choir: Arm with knowledge of disease prevention.
Soli: Condomize!
Choir: Arm with knowledge of disease prevention.
Soli: Vaccine!
Choir: Arm with knowledge of disease prevention.

C^{1}Soli S/A: If you use condom you will be safe.
Choir: Arm with knowledge of disease prevention.
S/A Call: If you use condom you'll be safe.
Choir: Arm with knowledge of disease prevention.

Recapitulation
B. Call: The nation must arm,
Resp: The nation must arm for the disease that is attacking us.
Call: The nation must arm,
Resp: The nation must arm for the disease that is attacking us.
Resp: The nation must arm for the disease that is attacking us.
Call: They must not arm with guns,
Resp: But with knowledge of disease prevention

According to Xolani, he, Phumlani, and Sizwe performed the song some years past with the composer, Obed Shangase. Section A of the original is left completely intact, though sometimes *uSomandla* 'God Almighty' is substituted for *uJesu* 'Jesus.'[1] In Section B, *makholwa* 'Christians' was replaced entirely with *Izizwe* 'the nation,' and *sathane* 'devil' was replaced with *isifo* 'disease, sickness.' The melody of sections C and C^1 were slightly musically altered. It ended with a recapitulation of section B.

The adaptation of this song conveys a feeling of ambiguity between the A section, with its Christological emphasis; however, the original song had a theme of struggle, which called for faith in the ever-present Jesus as a tool for fighting the devil. The same faith is in action here, for in the adaptation, the enemy is the devil in the form of the HIV; moreover, the choir has maintained that in the use of traditional and adapted gospel songs, in addition to their original numbers, local audiences connect with their message through recognizable musical forms.

MUSICAL QUOTATION

Quotation is a practice in the arts in which the creator of a piece of work pulls motivic material from a preexisting work and integrates it into the structural framework and development of a new artistic piece. In the visual arts, the practice is commonly known as parody (Hutcheon 1985). In the literary field, the model found expression in the Russian formalists' works, signaling a break of modernists from the Renaissance episteme (Hutcheon 1985: 2). In semiotic studies, the practice is more commonly called intertextuality (Bauman 2001; Bauman and Briggs 1992).

The practice of quotation in European polyphonic music has been commonplace for centuries, in several styles. The earliest, known from the ninth century onward and called *organum*, involves the parallel motion of voices against a quoted melody; in the fifteenth century, this texture, with the upper voices moving in a series of sixth-chords, became known as fauxbourdon. In a compositional process called *cantus-firmus* technique, first prominent in the late Middle Ages, a preexisting melody (*cantus prius factus*) is quoted note-for-note in one part, the tenor, which other voices envelop in counterpoint. In the style known as paraphrase, motifs in a reference melody are elaborated in counterpoint by all the voices. In the style known as parody, blocks of preexisting polyphony are quoted and elaborated (Reese 1959). Famously in the nineteenth century, Hector Berlioz (1803–1869) used the *cantus-firmus* technique in the fifth movement of his *Symphony Fantastique,* a section titled "Dream of a Witches' Sabbath." He quoted a medieval Gregorian chant, "Dies irae," the sequence sung after the *graduale* in the *missa defunctorum* (requiem mass) (*The Liber Usualis* 1963: 1810–1813). In measure 127 of the movement, the melody of the chant begins in the second trombones; tormenting motifs in the strings add counterpoint in insistent rhythms. By this combination of sounds, with the additional effects of the ringing of a bell, Berlioz invokes a sense of the grotesque.

In literary studies, parody or intertextuality serves the primary purpose of inscribing authors or speakers into their genre, letting them lay claim to the authority of canonical authenticity. In music, however, the practice of quotation can serve the purpose of inscribing meaning upon a performance by coopting a recognizable tune or passage from a previous musical event.

In African poetic performances such as epic pouring in Liberia, intertextuality is commonly employed to make a performance event relevant to the immediate audience through the deployment of recognizable thematic materials and delivery styles. For example, Kulung, the Kpelle epic pourer, conjures images and references which, though they may seem disjointed and unconnected to an audience from outside the tradition, nevertheless are recognizable and meaningful to his Kpelle audiences (Stone 2005: 56). Similarly in the Basotho migrants' song *lifela, the* cultural resources and political prestige of praise poetry (*lithoko*) is a backdrop to bring forth the migrants' experience: "long *lifela* contain images and passages donated by teachers or 'stolen' from other poets one has heard or competed with" (Coplan 1987: 431). By borrowing from one's teachers and poetic rivals, the *lifela* performer appropriates their experience and integrates them with his or hers, thus creating a spectrum of experience that is recognizably personal and at the same time general to the audience.

Siphithemba's music uses the quotation technique in two ways: in composition, and as a performance-delivery style. An example of quotation in composition is seen for instance in the song "Sizwile Ukuthi," (We've heard the gossip) by Sizwe Ndlela. In this song, Sizwe quoted the refrain of the Nguni wedding song "Ipi 'Ntombi Yam"[2] (Where's My Girl?), one of the signature soundtracks in the musical *Ipi Ntombi.*

A. Sizwile ukuthi thina bayasizonda
Kudumizwe lonke
Ukuthi thina sizenza ncono

B. *Soprano*: Higher, higher, oh we are going (2x)

C. *Alto*: Sinqamu lamazwe thina
Refrain: We are going, going higher and higher
Trio: Bayosala abanomona
Basala bekhuluma izindaba zabantu
Refrain: We are going, going higher and higher

D. *Sop Solo:* Bonke labantu (improvisation)
Refrain: Bayazithanda izindaba
Sop Solo: Bayazikhuluma izindaba
Refrain: Bayazikhuluma izindaba

A. We hear that they hate us
It's all over the world
That we have pride

B. Soprano: Higher, higher, oh we are going (2x)

C. Alto: We go all places
Refrain: We are going, going higher and higher
Trio: We leave the jealous
We leave them talking about us
Refrain: We are going, going higher and higher

D. Sop Solo: All of them
Refrain: They love news [gossiping]
Sop Solo: They are gossiping
Refrain: They are gossiping

In performing this song, the choir clearly deploys language and gestural devices to send a taunting message to an intended audience who are perceived to be in some form of contestation with them. In section A, rendered in IsiZulu, the choir members place right or left hands to their ears, gesturing that they are hearing rumors or gossip going around about them. Section B is in English, and is a linguistic adaptation and musical quotation from the musical soundtrack. The original tune sang *haya, haya o intombi yam,* where *haya, haya* is merely vocables, with no specific meaning. In composing this song, Sizwe adapted the sound to English as *higher, higher,* but with an assertive sense of motion and teleology. The singers gesture an upward pointing of the first fingers, signifying their higher movement. Section C is set to an overlapping call-and-response pattern, forming a dialogic process between the alto and trio call lines, sung in Zulu, and the repeated choral refrain line, sung in English. This section is performed to a dance movement that mimics ambling motion. The D section returns completely to the Zulu language and is performed to a series of movements as the section continues to repeat. The last two dance movements include counterclockwise movement. Here, gestures are adapted from children's plays, in which young girls taunt boys or their peers by placing their hands on their hips and wiggling their waists sideways. In performing the section, the choir members place their left hands on their hips, wiggling them sideways while their right hands make gestures resembling military salutes. In the last dance form, the choir members stand in a semicircle, stretching out their arms in a gesture that mimics the riding of motorbikes. They sing a full round of the section while turning gradually, first to the right and moving their shoulders up and down in rhythm. The right foot is raised to a slight stamp to close the final cadence of the round. The cycle is repeated again in the leftward direction, with the final cadence closing with a slight stamp of the left foot. This process is repeated several times, until the leading soloist signals for a stop by slowing down on the last call with a *molto ritardando.* In South Africa, the rhythmic shoulder-motion gesture often signifies a joyous state, and therefore is celebratory, especially where the jubilant is perceived to have defied all odds to achieve success.

But, what is the purpose of this song, and why the technic of musical quotation in the composition? Upon hearing this song, I became filled with curiosity. I wondered what the choir was celebrating and who was gossiping about them. In short, who is the intended audience? According to Sizwe, he

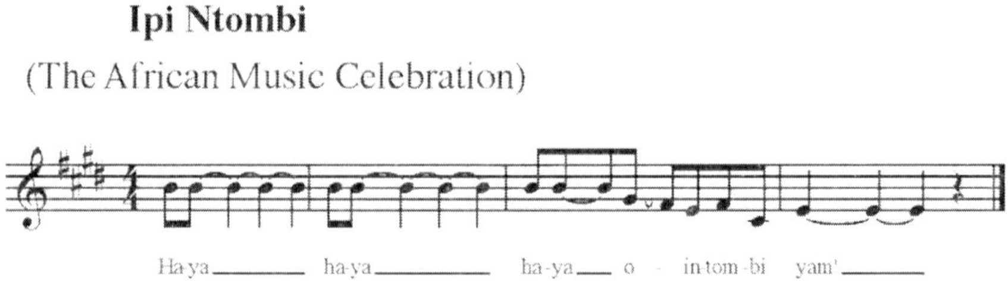

Figure 6.1 Transcription of the refrain of "Ipi Intombi."

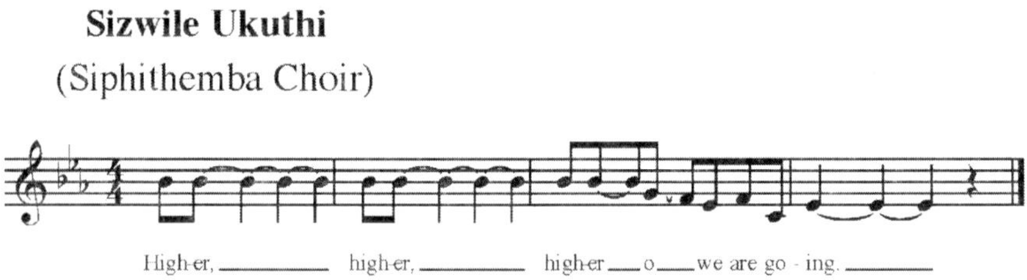

Figure 6.2 Siphithemba's Quotation of the "Ipi Intombi" refrain.

composed the song upon return from the Tenth Retroviruses and Opportunistic Infections Conference in Boston. He however was not forthcoming in explaining what had informed his writing of the song. His initial response to my question as to why he wrote the song was general and vague. According to him, "when people know that you are HIV-positive, they don't think that you can do anything. But when they see us doing things, and going to places, then they wonder and say 'Ah, ah, how come?'"

Phakamile, Nomusa, and Mrs. Mhlongo gave more detailed accounts of events that informed the song. First, McCord Hospital, like many health institutions that cater mainly to the Black community in the Greater Durban and Ngungundlovu areas, has standing staff choirs. In fact, the McCord Nurses Choir is about the oldest hospital staff choir in the area, and probably among the oldest in all of South Africa. In chapter 2 of this work, I indicated that Katie Makanya, who would later become Dr. McCord's medical assistant, was among the African Jubilee Singers from the Eastern Cape who had toured Great Britain. Conversations with the medical superintendent, Dr. Holst, indicated that Katie is believed to have been part of the effort to start the nurses' choir at the hospital in the early days; hence, the choir was the hospital's artistic image-maker until the Siphithemba Choir came on the scene.

From 1997, much of the hospital's public-relations initiatives, health-awareness campaigns, and fund drives, were HIV/AIDS-related. Hence, it made sense to showcase the Siphithemba Choir in all these efforts. With the

HIV/AIDS project, the management and outside dignitaries visiting the hospital paid more attention to the Sinikithemba Support Group and the choir than to the staff choir. All accounts from the hospital management and those of the choir suggest that the choir was treated like a pearl in the heart of the hospital. Apparently, this resulted in ill-feelings between the Siphithemba Choir and the staff choir—feelings that became heightened when the Siphithemba Choir began making trips overseas. Some support group and choir members recall overhearing some hospital staff make cynical remarks about the choir members who now enjoyed "the privilege of traveling to America"—a privilege they would never have dreamed about, "just because they are HIV-positive." Such remarks certainly contained ironies, in that they were sick patients being cared for by the nurses and staff of the hospital. Theirs was previously a state of hopelessness, wherein neither they nor their caregivers imagined that they would survive much longer.

Another conflict occurred within the choir itself. During its first tour of the United States, in 2002, sponsored by the Church World Services, the ensemble had about forty voices, but when Professor Bruce Walker invited them to the Tenth Conference on Retroviruses and Opportunistic Infections in Boston, in 2003, he could sponsor only twenty. Phumlani and Mrs. Mhlongo had to use an auditioning process to screen the number down, making room for the "best" twenty singers. The process generated resentment on the part of members who thought they were being eliminated unfairly. Phumlani was caught in the middle of the controversy—which prompted Mrs. Mhlongo to bring in independent choral conductors to complete the auditioning process.

In the course of preparations to travel to Boston, Clover, a Durban-based diary company, which produced sour milk, held an AIDS awareness-education campaign as part of its corporate social program and public-relations initiative. The company enlisted the Siphithemba Choir to promote its program. The invitation was nearly turned down by the hospital, since it coincided with the choir's trip to Boston, but Mrs. Mhlongo suggested that those who had been screened out of the touring group could constitute another choir to perform at the event. Unfortunately this move resulted in an acrimonious division within the support group and the choir, wherein the two groups constituted themselves into cliques pitched against each other.

In Zulu, sour milk is called *amasi*, a delicacy that is now mostly associated with the rural and poor township dwellers in present-day KwaZulu-Natal. The group that was billed to travel to Boston began referring to the alternate group as *Kwayaamasi* 'Sour Milk Choir' and called themselves the "Overseas Choir." Hence, when Sizwe and the "Overseas Choir" premiered the song shortly upon return from Boston, the alternate group took offense about it.

From Nomusa's and Phakamile's account, Mrs. Mhlongo was equally upset about the song.

Later on, Sizwe acknowledged to me that the issue between the alternate groups had been a factor that partly informed his composition of the piece. Conversations with other choir members showed that the controversy that the song had generated among the members of the Sinikithemba Support Group had prompted another intervention from Mrs. Mhlongo. From all these interviews and conversations, I could deduce that the more general meaning about the song as speaking to those who stigmatize people living with AIDS was a later interpretation, designed to mitigate the tension brewing between the groups. When I pressed Mrs. Mhlongo for her interpretation of the song, she carefully avoided linking the song to the conflict in the group by responding in general terms: "You know, people like members to disclose their status, and yet they don't disclose [*their own status*] themselves." This signaled for me the effort by participants in the story of the Siphithemba Choir to maintain a positive image of the group and not let their internal differences derail their goal of bringing the message of hope to the members and their communities.

In subsequent trips overseas, the number of members was expanded to about thirty voices, but acrimony between the groups did not cease. For an immigration-related reason, Mrs. Mhlongo did not attend the international conference in Boston, where she had been billed to give the keynote address on behalf of the AIDS project at McCord Hospital.[3] Zinhle, a choir member and participant in the trial of the antiretroviral therapy, gave the address in her place. In South Africa, Mrs. Mhlongo ended up going to the Clover event with the alternate choir. It is unclear whether she developed some special bonding with the alternate group as a result of these events, but from her testimony when administrative and procedural issues led to her resignation from her post a year or so later, a large section of the support group left with her, including almost all of the members of the alternate choir group, while the "Overseas Choir" remained with the hospital.

The choir continued to perform "Sizwile Ukuthi" on different occasions since then, almost certainly suppressing its original meaning. They now use it to convey a sense of resilience and determination to overcome the perceived odds of being HIV-positive. Choir members attest to the fact that their families, friends, and neighbors have become more and more receptive and respectful of them since they began touring overseas. Without a doubt, I observed that members of the choir exuded more confidence and pride than members of other support groups that I encountered during the course of this research. The singing, the emotional stability, the international exposure and affirmation, and material success that they have achieved are largely responsible for their sense of confidence and pride.

In another compositional practice, Siphithemba engages in self-parody by quoting motivic or thematic materials of one of their songs in another. An example is the quotation of part of original song "Know Your Status," (see appendix) composed by Phumlani, with contributions from other choir members in the adaption of the gospel song "Izizwe Mazihlome" (full lyrics already provided in chapter 4). In this song, the choir quotes section C of "Know Your Status," and then layers the solo calls "abstain," "be faithful," and "condomize" over the section C of "Izizwe Mazihlome." Meanwhile, the soprano solo retains her calls, which demand that the nation must not arm with actual war implements, such as guns or spears, while the choir responds with "[but] arm with knowledge of disease prevention." With each constituent part singing lyrical and melodic contents that are different from the rest, while maintaining a unifying tonal center, what is heard is overlapping call and response,

C. Sop. Solo: Zingahlomi ngezibhamu bo;
Soli: Abstain!
Choir: Zihlome ngolwazi lokuvikele ubhubhane.

Sop. Solo: Zingahlomi ngemikhonto bo;
Soli: Be faithful!
Choir: Zihlome ngolwazi lokuvikele ubhubhane.

Sop. Solo: Zingahlomi ngezibhamu bo;
Soli: Condomize!
Choir: Zihlome ngolwazi lokuvikele ubhubhane.

Sop. Solo: Zingahlomi ngemikhonto bo;
Soli: Vaccine!
Choir: Zihlome ngolwazi lokuvikele ubhubhane.

[C. Sop. Solo: They must not arm with guns;
Soli: Abstain!
Choir: Arm with knowledge of disease prevention.
Sop. Solo: They must not arm with spears;
Soli: Be faithful!
Choir: Arm with knowledge of disease prevention.

Sop. Solo: They must not arm with guns;
Soli: Condomize!
Choir: Arm with knowledge of disease prevention.

Sop. Solo: They must not arm with spears;
Soli: Vaccine!
Choir: Arm with knowledge of disease prevention.

In yet another form of quotation, Siphithemba takes a section of a preexisting song and merges it with a section of another song, thereby making an unsuspecting audience hear them as one piece. I wish to revisit two songs that have already been analyzed in chapter 5, "Isiyalo" (Advice) and "Ikhalaphi" (From Hence the Cry) (see full song texts in chapter 5) here by examining how these two songs have been performed by the Choir and how the performance practice helps to reinforce the meaning and the intended message the choir seeks to convey.

Clearly, the two songs are different, and Siphithemba has performed them separately. But on several occasions, the choir omitted the opening section of "Ikhalaphi" and instead merged the second part with "Isiyalo." A close reading shows that the B section of "Ikhalaphi" actually reinforces the message in "Isiyalo." In traditional Zulu society, a girl should remain a virgin until marriage. As stated in chapter 3, the current Zulu monarch, Nkosi Zwelithini, has tried to uphold and to preserve this value through the institution of the reed dance (also called umNkosi woMhlaba), in which young girls moving into womanhood present reed sticks to the king.

KwaMasonto, as referenced in the song, most likely hails from a dysfunctional home, where she has no good advice, travels across the hills (probably to the city), and engages in "twenty-cent games" (prostitution). The reference to her rejecting the marriage proposal is a misnomer, for in actuality, by the standards of Zulu traditional values, KwaMasonto is no longer fit for marriage.

Musically, a slight disjuncture occurs in the transition in tempo and rhythm, because "Isiyalo" is performed in a simple quadruple time (4/4), but the second section of "Ikhalaphi" is performed to compound quadruple time (12/8). It is not uncommon in African music for tempo, rhythm, or even time signature to change to suit certain accompanying dances or strengthen the message being conveyed, or both. In this style of quotation music, the slight disjoint is minimized by the continuity in dance. Once the second section of "Ikhalaphi" is started, the choreographed dance is replaced with the folk style of the *ukusina,* wherein the choristers use ululations and hand gestures to challenge one another to come forward and demonstrate their facility with the dance. At this juncture, anybody in the audience—man, woman, or child—is free to join in the performance by coming to the front and making the dance moves. I observed that audience participation in this dance happens only when the choir performs in Black townships or rural areas where Black people exclusively constitute the event community. Black townships still have a sense that a musical performance is a communal event, in which boundaries between audience and performers are blurred.

At all performances before a racially mixed audience in urban settings, the choir performs this piece alone. In urban centers, especially in racially mixed

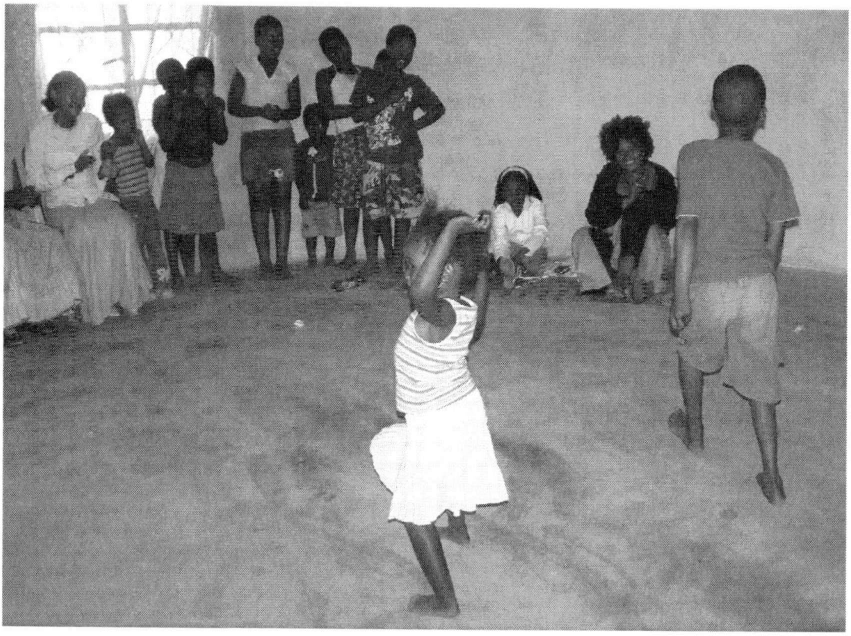

Figure 6.3 A little girl demonstrates the Zulu dance.

gatherings, the Western dichotomy of performers and audience is very much observed. Upon inquiry, all choir members agreed that the people who make up the audience in the townships and rural communities understand the nature of the song and dance, and the fact that every male or female present is not only free to join in the dance but is in fact expected to come forward to do the dance.

Again, quotation enables performers to draw from materials that are recognizable to their immediate audience. But in this form of quotation, drawing from a recognizable traditional song not only helps the audience appreciate the meaning embedded in the song through the lens of cultural knowledge, but signals for them when the music event has broken from the rigid dichotomy of performer and audience, and ushers in the familiar scene of active participation by all, which characterizes the communality of a typical African music event.

SERMONETTES AND SHORT PRAYER FORMULARY

As indicated in my discussion of gospel music above, South African gospel artists perceive themselves to be engaged in the ministry of preaching the

Christian gospel through their music. Many artists accomplish this goal by inserting short declamatory forms of preaching called sermonette and/or short prayer formularies within songs. Sermonette according to Portia Maultsby is the ad-lib vocal gestures that gospel artists use to establish rapport with their audience (2005: 329). I use the term in this work to designate similar practice in South African gospel singing. The choir has no word for the practice, although in South Africa, the practice functions exactly the way it does in African American gospel. Sermonettes also reinforce the message embedded in a specific song, such as a personal relationship with God, repudiation of sin and rejection of Satan, salvation and peace with God, and eschatological vision. Hence Siphithemba members view themselves as a gospel choir. They preach the gospel through their music and organizational activities, which encapsulate the spirituality of hope and faith in God in the presence of HIV and AIDS. Their songs are sermonic, in that they declare a state of emergency using the kerygmatic formula, as in their song "Siyaphela isizwe seNkosi" (The Nation of the Lord Is Finishing). They encourage their audience to look unto God as source of hope and strength, as in "Izizwe Mazihlome" (The Nation Must Arm); they demand of people to test as in "You've got to Know Your Status," and they point out the root of the problem in "Isiyalo" (Advice) and "Ikhalaphi" (From Whence the Cry).

In specific Siphithemba song examples, sermonettes are sometimes paired with a short prayer formulary. What one hears is prayer with an underlying sermonic message. The song "Jehovah," composed jointly by Phumlani, Zinhle, Sizwe, and Xolani, illustrates this phenomenon.

Jehovah

Jehovah, Jehovah,
Qhawe elikhulu ngonyama yezwe

Sikhala kuwe,
Sinxusa kuwe,
Siphe amandla,
Sinqoba izilingo.

Prayer formulary

Kulonhlaba esiphila kuwo,
Ocwele izilingo,
Oh Nkosi kungani sibulalana sodwa?
Kungani kubulawa izingane ezingakafiki kulomhlaba?
Sithi baba,
Yehlisa amandla akho;

Ngoba ngaphandle kwakho,
Ngeke senza lutho.

Trio: Ngonyama yamazulu,
Qhawe lamaqhawe,
Ungumfeli waboni bomhlaba,
Sihawukele thina boni.

Bheka, sididekile,
Asazi nokuthi kwenzekani.
Sibona igazi liphalala;
Oh kungenxa yamacala ethu.
Solo: Siyakhala phambi kwakho,

Refrain: Sikhala kuwe,
Sinxusa kuwe,
Siphe amandla,
Okunqoba izilingo.

Jehovah, Jehova,
You're the great hero of the black nation

We cry to you,
We plead you,
Give us power,
To conquer temptations.

Prayer formulary

In this world,
full of temptations,
Oh Lord why do we kill each other?
Why do we kill the unborn babies?
We say to you father,
Give us your power;
Because without you,
There is nothing we can do.

Trio: King of heaven,
Lord of lords,
You died for our sins,
Have mercy on us sinners.

See, we don't know what to do,

We don't know what is happening.
We see bloodshed;
Oh, it's because of our sins.

Solo: We cry in your presence,

Refrain: We cry to you,
We beg you,
Give us power,
To conquer temptations.

This song opens with a theme that speaks of Black Nationalism, by referring to God as "the great hero of the black nation" (an issue that I will address in detail in chapter 7). But in the overall scheme, the song is a prayer that asks God to intervene in the face of the problem. There is recognition of the powerlessness of the people and their community, and a verbal act of prostration before God as the omnipotent who alone can salvage the situation by helping them conquer temptations. The formulary usually delivered by Xolani over a choral humming of the refrain reinforces the theme of the song, which is a petition for power to overcome temptations. But the prayer opens by declaring, "this world is full of temptations." Then it appears to interrogate the rationale for all the "homicides" and "abortions," but that is not quite the case. The sermonette part of the song must not be construed as merely speaking about homicide and abortion, for in Phumlani's words,

> When we think about the fact that sometimes people know that they are HIV-positive, but they refuse to tell their partner, then you have unprotected sex with her, and if she becomes pregnant, then the baby can also become positive, you see, so anytime I do that, I actually put the innocent child in danger, and this is part of the problem.

In another song, "Friendship with Jesus," Nomusa declares a prayer layered over the humming of the refrain. The prayer points to steadfastness with God, in spite of having lost loved ones to AIDS.

Friendship with Jesus
Duet: There is no other name,
There is no other love, theory
Except Jesus.

Refrain
Solo: Friendship with Jesus,

Chorus: Friendship with Jesus;
Fellowship with Jesus;
Solo: Divine oh Lord;
What a blessed sweet communion,
Jesus is the friend of mine.

Refrain is repeated to a humming with short prayer delivered by Nomusa thus:
Heavenly Father we pray,
As we are gathered here dear God praising your name,
Nowadays dear Lord, we are faced with this disease HIV and AIDS.
And we have lost our loved ones dear God,
But even so we are still praising your name.
And we are asking you dear Lord,
We are begging you,
That you may please,
Please dear God,
Give us the cure. Amen

Refrain and close

The prayer formulary does not directly reinforce the theme of the song, since the song does not speak directly about HIV/AIDS. Nevertheless, the prayer brings the theme of relationship with God to the fore by emphasizing that they gather to praise God's name, even when they have lost loved ones. This is an indication of their commitment to relationship with God; in spite the odds and burdens of HIV and AIDS. The song underscores their faith and the hope they have in God's graciousness and omnipotence.

FORM AND STRUCTURE IN SIPHITHEMBA SONGS

I use the term *form* loosely in this work, because Siphithemba songs have thematic sections that are either melodically or lyrically informed, and that therefore give the songs perceivable formal structures. In my analyses, I use the A–B–C–D style to represent the segments of each song, but that does not necessarily mean they correspond to Western classical forms.

Many characteristic features of the ensemble's music can be analyzed, but that would entail carrying out analysis of all the songs in their repertory—which would exceed the scope of this work. My aim here is to isolate the most important and specific traits of their music, to illustrate that Siphithemba and their music reflect a continuity, rather than a shift, in the South African—nay, Zulu—choral-music tradition. For example, David K. Rycroft observed about Zulu indigenous singing as being antiphonal in form with at least two voice parts singing non-identical texts performed to leader–chorus call-and-response and overlapping phrases—which gives rise to polyphony (1977:222). This style of singing creates a cyclic loop, wherein individual participants could interject their own voices and texts almost independently of, but in sonorous relationship to the two main parts, thus creating heterophony. Another is the structural styles that characterize Enoch Sontonga's and John Knox Bokwe's masterworks that have influenced Black South African choral tradition. Both Enoch Sontonga's "Nkosi Sikelele iAfrika" and John Knox Bokwe's "Plea for Africa" exhibit a conscious integration of Western homophonic hymn style (in measures 1–10) with the African-derived call-and-response technique (in measures 11–15). Zulu indigenous polyphonic singing, and the early composers' combination of Western homophonic hymn style with African call-response techniques, characterizes much of Siphithemba's songs. Most of their gospel songs replicate the structure of Enoch Sontonga's "Nkosi Sikelele iAfrika" and John Knox Bokwe's "Plea for Africa." This structure consists of two major sections, where the first section usually presents a four-part homophonic texture, often rendered in declamatory style, and the second section presents any of several call-and-response textures involving a soloist and the choir, or two or more different vocal parts.

In some of Siphithemba's songs, the opening section could begin with a solo call, but the section is still set to four-part homophonic singing, while the subsequent section is set to extensive overlapping calls and responses. Siphithemba songs have subsections within the bisectional framework. The following songs of Siphithemba replicate this structure: "Siyakubonga Somandla" (We Thank You, God); "Sizwile Ukuthi" (We've Heard the Gossip); "Jehova"; "Izizwe Mazihlome" (The Nation Must Arm); "Lalelani" (Listen); "Siyaphela isizwe seNkosi" (The Nation of the Lord Is Finishing); "Know Your Status"; and "Ngizohamba" (I'm Going). One song, "Know Your Status" (see appendix) effectively illustrates this musical phenomenon.

A

a

You've go to know your status

We all know our status. (3x)

b

If negative, stay negative.

If positive, think positive. (3x)

B

c

Abstain!

Be faithful! (3x)

Condomize!

d

Sop: Take your medicine. (3x)

Choir: Even if you're feeling better. (*layered over the sopranos*)

Noma usuzizwa uphila

(*Even if—and Noma usuzizwa is alternated in part-counter-part form*)

This song has two four internal a-b-c-d segments, embedded in a larger two-part structure A-B, performed to a soundtrack. The A section is performed in homophonic chord progression and is declamatory in nature. In fact, the choir adds emphasis to the declamation with hand gestures that challenge the audience to know their status. In the B section, the c segment begins by laying down the ABC rules (Abstain, Be faithful, Condomize). First, all voices sing "abstain, be faithful" three times, and then the males layer their own melody of "condomize" over the females, who hold onto "abstain, be faithful." The males accompany their singing with hand gesture that suggests the putting on of condoms. This is repeated thrice before they transition to the *d* segment, which begins with a soprano voice introducing "take your medicine," to which the choir responds "even if you're feeling better" and "noma usuzizwa uphila" all at the same time. The Zulu phrase *noma usuzizwa uphila* 'even if you're feeling better' already signals the beginning of multiple text renditions in the music. Thenceforth, the choir splits into seven different parts, all singing different melodies and different texts at the same time but with a perceivable dialogic sequence, and without any tincture of dissonance. The style of singing in multiple texts and multi-part dialogic sequence corresponds to what Olly Wilson (1992) termed "heterogeneous sound ideal" in African music. According to Wilson, the heterogeneous sound ideal is realized by a complex mosaic interaction of lead voice, chorus, and instruments (1992: 331–332), being also sonic manipulation of individual and group experiences of life and of the spiritual world as social dynamic (see Floyd 1995: 32).

Ruth Stone found similar dialogic-style performance in her study of Kpelle epic pouring (2004: 72–73); she described the complex layering of voices as a dialogue or transaction in pairs, among the voices in the performance

(2004: 73). In the pairing, one could contrast the soloist to the song catcher, the song catcher and chorus, and the soloist and the chorus. If the performing parts are labeled XYZ, the pairing of performers would be heard as X⇔Y and Y⇔Z and X⇔Z. In my own analysis of the song under study, this form of pairing could be heard in the following way: Sop. Solo ⇔ Sop. I/II/Alto I/Countertenor/Baritone for the first layer of dialogic interaction. The second layer of dialogic interaction is heard thus: Alto II/Countertenor ⇔Sop. I/II/ Alto I/Baritone.

Examined in the light of Zulu worldview, the dialogic style of musical performance articulates with the sense of community at two levels. First, the Zulu social world can be described as a bifilar system, underscored often by gender compartmentalization. The bifilar gender-compartmentalized social world is typified in an observation I made while attending ritual events in rural areas with members of the Siphithemba Choir. Upon entering any house, men sit on the right from the entrance door, separate from women and children, who sit on the left (see figure 6.4). The same pattern is observable upon entering homesteads. The man's hut is located on the right side of the entrance, and his wife (or wives) and children's hut(s) stand on the left, facing the man's. Also, just as the songs are set in dialogic relationships and rendered in repetitive cyclic form, the huts and the homesteads are built around or in a circle. The men and women with children are placed in opposite directions—a dialogic form of relationships. This observable social world structure that found expression in music is not new. In fact there is evidence of this in early missionary documentations. A certain Lady Pinkerton for example described this social world in a nascent mission church in the 1870s in her journal thus:

> I have just returned from a service in the chapel, and think you will be interested in a description of the building, and of the people who worship there every Sunday. The chapel was built by Rev. Mr. Stone, who lived here twenty years. . . . The roof is thatched; but there is no ceiling. Next to the thatches are the heavy beams not smooth and painted, but rough, just as they were taken from the woods. . . . But our attention is called to those who occupy these benches every Sabbath. On one side are the men, on the other the women. (1870: 337[4])

Lady Pinkerton has an elaborate description of the design of this house, but does not say what geometric shape it has, yet it is possible that the building was round, given that Zulu thatches—roof made from grass or straw are designed round. The sitting arrangement in the chapel, with men and women on opposite sides, shows that the Zulu were already using their indigenous cultural forms to transform the space of the mission church to fit with their own cultural ideals, a practice that has persisted in much of postcolonial and post-apartheid Zulu society.

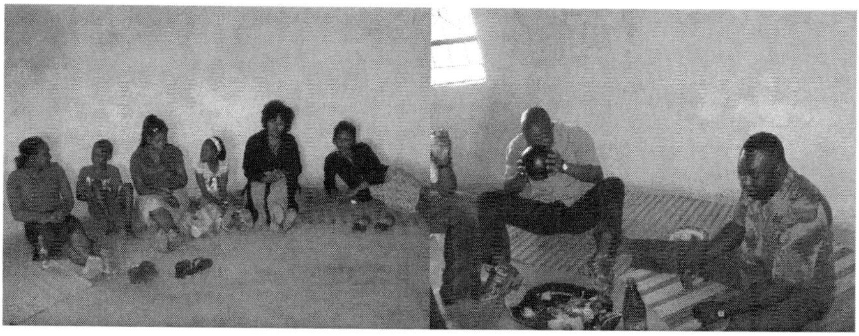

Figure 6.4 Sitting arrangement in a Zulu round house.

The second is the sense of *indaba* as an integral component of the *ubuntu* philosophy. In chapter 5, I explained the concept of *indaba* as a dialogic process in which competing and/or complementing parties engage to resolve or prevent emergent crises in the community. In such a process, the parties involved share a common agenda—that of realizing a cohesive social system, in which everyone has a stake. Musically speaking, the cohesion is made possible by the ability of each constituent part in the choral performance to maintain the tonal center irrespective of lyrical or melodic differences from the rest of the choir. A close attention to the tonal center helps each soloist and vocal part achieve consonant harmonic effect, even when extensive improvisations occur.

INSTRUMENTATION AND DANCE

The Siphithemba Choir uses different styles of instrumentation to accompany their singing when it is paired with dance. Here I want to describe the two main types of dance as they relate to the instrumentation that accompanies their singing.

Siphithemba's instrumentation styles are divided according to the two genres of choral singing that make up their repertory: traditional songs and gospel songs. The traditional songs can be accompanied with Zulu drums (*idlamu*) and handclapping, to correspond with the foot-stamping of the *ukusina* dance. Because of the controversy over the *idlamu* (explained in chapter 7) and the choir's effort to mitigate any rift with the hospital management, the choir now accompanies most of its traditional songs with only handclapping; however, at some events the choir does not hesitate to turn any useful object within reach into an instrument to provide rhythmic accompaniment.

A second type of instrumentation is of soundtracks. The choir owns an electric bass, a drum set, a synthesizer keyboard, amplifiers, and speakers. These are part of the ensemble of instruments that are used by gospel artists in South Africa, just like their American counterparts. But Siphithemba uses these only during choir rehearsals, never for performances. The cost of transporting these instruments for local or international tours would be prohibitive; hence the decision to produce sound tracks to accompany the choir's gospel songs. In the absence of the use of the *idlamu,* the choir developed instrumental soundtracks also for some of their traditional repertoire.

In my conversations with Xolani, I learned that the idea of using prerecorded instrumental music to accompany the choir's gospel songs came from the practice that is already in place in South Africa among several gospel choirs. Some gospel choirs and artists tend to perform songs by African American gospel artists, especially within church worship or at concert events. Renowned artists who have their own bands with skilled musicians can reproduce the original sound of the American artists. Others resort to purchasing the instrumental soundtrack versions of the original recording, and then sing over the prerecorded tracks. It has become a common practice among gospel artists and even popular artists to use prerecorded tracks at concerts where they have no accompanying band of their own.

CHOREOGRAPHED AND NONCHOREOGRAPHED DANCE

Almost all of Siphithemba's songs are integrated with dance. Since most of their gospel songs are performed over prerecorded soundtracks, the accompanying dance forms are choreographed to fit the rhythm and the formal structure of the recordings. Similarly, in the absence of Zulu drums, the choir has created its own prerecorded sound tracks to accompany its traditional songs, using instruments such as the electric bass, drum sets, and a synthesizer keyboard. Hence the traditional Zulu songs, which would usually be improvised within *ukusina* dance style, are now performed with choreographed movements.

Few songs in the choir's traditional repertoire are performed without prerecorded soundtracks. Those that are not accompanied with soundtracks include "Ikhalaphi" (From Whence the Cry), "Seliyaduma" (It's Thundering), and "Hamba Lulu" (Go Lulu). Although "Nkonyane kaNdaba" (Son of Ndaba) is not performed to prerecorded tracks, the accompanying dance is still choreographed. Other traditional pieces are performed over soundtracks with accompanying choreographed dances. These include "Isiyalo" (Advice), "Mama, Ndiyagoduka Ngomso" (Mama, I'm Going Home Tomorrow), and "Ibonakala Nganina?" (How Does She Show She loves Him?).

Siphithemba uses three categories of movements in its choreographed dances: symbolic bodily gestures, which express the meanings of the sung texts; nonsymbolic bodily gestures, which often fall on instrumental interludes; and *ukusina* dance, used in the traditional songs.

I will use "Isiyalo" to illustrate the use of these categories of gestures. For the sake of visual clarity, these descriptions are thus summarized in a table.

Section A

Table 6.1 "Isiyalo," words, movements, and gestural meanings of section A

Music and sung text	*Accompanying movement/ gesture*	*Meaning*
Instrumental Introduction	No gesture	None
Solo: *Asikho isiyalo la izalwakhona* 'There's no advice from whence she comes'	Singer points randomly in any direction	Accusation/indictment of the subject in the song
Choir: *Asikho isiyalo la izalwakhona* 'There's no advice from whence she comes'	Singers swing two hands up & down. They drop their arms at the downbeats, and the two hands cross at the upbeat	Negative sign to show that the subject in the song has no good upbringing
Iphum' ekhaya 'She comes from home'	No gesture	None
Igqoke kahle 'She is dressed up'	Both palms open, down-to-up-down hand motion	Subject is dressed up
Ifike ngalena kwendaba 'She comes across the hills'	Both palms open & facing forward; singers make a down-to-up-down hand motion	Subject traverses the hills
Ekumule idilozi ilibeke phansi 'She strips pants and puts it down'	Singers stoop and make a downward hand motion from the hips	Subject strips
Thubhobho i-gemu 'For a 20-cent game'	Still stooping, singers show the index and middle fingers, alternating between both hands	Subject collects 20c (1 = 10) + (1 = 10) = 20 from here & there—an act of prostitution
Asikho isiyalo la izalwakhona 'There's no advice from whence she comes'	Singers swing both hands up & down. They drop their arms at the downbeats and the two hands cross up at the upbeat	Negative sign to show that the subject in the song has no good upbringing
Instrumental interlude; rhythmic change	No gesture	None

The second part of the song, following the interlude, is set to call-and-response form. The lead solo calls *ayivumi ngishela kwaMasondo ayivumi,* and the choir responds with *ngishela kwaMasondo ayivumi,* and immediately the response forms a cyclic loop of responses to the lead soloist. He calls *ayivumi ngishela kwaMasondo ayivumi* twice, and *le'ntombi yenzani* four times while he keeps dancing in front of the choir. He repeats the cycle, and then dances at the edge of the line in the third cycle.

Section B
1st, 2nd, & 3rd cycles:

Table 6.2 "Isiyalo," words, movements, and gestural meanings of section B, cylcles 1, 2, and 3

Music and sung text	*Accompanying movement or gesture*	*Meaning*
Solo: Ayivumi ngishela kwaMasondo ayivumi 'She rejects my proposal'	Singer points randomly in any direction	Accusation or indictment of the subject in the song
Choir: Ngishela kwaMasondo ayivumi 'I propose [to] kwaMasondo; she refuses'	Singers wind both arms in front, and then move them backward to the sides, with open arms facing forward	Subject KwaMasondo despises the marriage proposal
Solo: Le'ntombi yenzani? 'What is the young lady doing?'	Singer points randomly in any direction	Accusation or indictment of the subject in the song
Choir: Ngishela kwaMansondo ayivumi 'I propose [to] kwaMasondo; she refuses'	Singers wind both arms in front, and then move them backward to the sides, with open arms facing forward	Subject KwaMasondo despises the marriage proposal

In the fourth, fifth, and sixth cycles, the choir breaks into two groups of two different dance movements. One group maintains the hand gestures indicating kwaMasonto's refusal of the marriage proposal, while a second group performs a choreographed form of *ukusina* and *phatha phatha*[5] dances. The two groups alternate in the movements. The first group, consisting of up to four singers, dances forward to eight measured steps, corresponding with the refrain, while making the *ukunyakazisa* gesture (shaking of the hands in imitation of the brandishing of a spear), and then stamping the feet first on the third beat of the second round of the refrain, beginning with the right foot, to the rhythm of a dotted quarter note, plus a left foot-stamp to the value of an eighth note tied to a quarter note on the downbeat of the next measure. They stamp the right and left feet to even quarter notes on the second and

ISIYALO

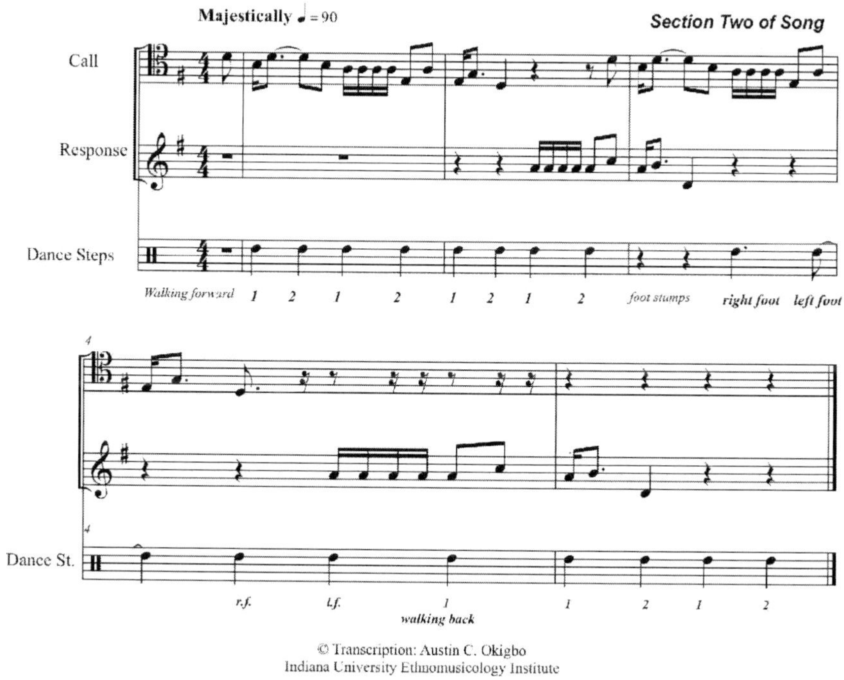

Figure 6.5 Traditional Zulu song with accompanying dance steps.

third beats respectively, and then return to the line by walking backward, starting with the number one in the upbeat of the second measure of the round of refrain, only to reach the line at the final cadence of the round (see figure 6.5).

Section B
4th, 5th, & 6th cycles

Closing cycle to fade
Working with Siphithemba marked the only instance in the course of this research that I found a group combining choreographed elements of traditional dance with modern dance styles and Western-style instrumental production. This was an innovation that had come out of necessity in the absence of the Zulu drums. By doing so, however, the choir succeeded to a great extent in retaining the traditional elements of their music in the circumstances of necessity and innovation.

Table 6.3 "Isiyalo," Section B, cycles 4, 5, and 6, words, movements, and gestural meanings.

Music and sung text	*Accompanying movement or gesture*	*Meaning*
Solo: Ayivumi ngishela kwaMasondo ayivumi 'She rejects my proposal to kwaMasondo'	Group of singers dance 8 measured steps forward	None
Choir: Ngishela kwaMasondo ayivumi 'I propose [to] kwaMasondo; she refuses'	Group of singers take 3 consecutive right foot and 1 left foot ukusina stamp	Traditional dance choreographed
Solo: Le'ntombi yenzani? (4x) 'What is the young lady doing?' (4x)"	Group of singers dance 8 measure steps back to original position, crossing a second group halfway	None
Ngishela kwaMansondo ayivumi 'I propose [to] kwaMasondo; she refuses'	Group of singers dance 8 measured steps forward	None
	Group of singers pat their hips to the right and to the left	phatha phata dance choreographed
	Group of singers throw up left, and then right hands and leap as they do so	None
	Group of singers dance 8 measured steps back to original position	None

Table 6.4 Closing cycle of "Isiyalo" to fade.

Solo: Ayivumi ngishela kwaMasondo ayivumi 'She rejects my proposal to kwaMasondo'	All singers retake original position in single line	None
Choir: Ngishela kwaMasondo ayivumi 'I propose [to] kwaMasondo; she refuses (2x)	Singers stretch out arms sideways and swing back and forth sideways while shaking their hands	None
Solo: Le'ntombi yenzani? 'What is the young lady doing?' (4x)		
Ngishela kwaMansondo ayivumi 'I propose [to] kwaMasondo; she refuses'	Ditto	None
	Ditto	None

SINGING AND DANCING THE MEETING

Toward the end of my extended stay in Durban and work with the Siphithemba Choir, the group organized a surprise farewell party for me on a Sunday afternoon at the home of Phakamile and her sister Wicky in Umlazi. They had tricked me into coming to the event by suggesting that Nomusa's family was holding an *umsebenzi,* hoping that this would be an attraction for me. The representatives of the U.S. President's Emergency Plan for AIDS Relief (PEPFAR) were visiting McCord Hospital that week. Martin Freeth, the managing director of the Windfall Digital Film Company from the United Kingdom, was there with his crew to document activities at the hospital for PEPFAR, and they had asked to meet with Siphithemba Choir on the same Sunday.

I quickly went home after mass at the Emmanuel Cathedral, got my equipment ready, and headed to the Cato Crest to pick up Ncamisile and her two kids. Then we passed by the Durban CBD to pick up Sizile. I asked Ncamisile how the choir intended to handle the film crew for the PEPFAR project at the same time as the *umsebenzi* would be going on, but she said, "I don't know; we'll see." Ncamisile then announced that we had to pass through Umlazi to pick up Phakamile, Wicky, and Phakamile's son before we could head off to Nomusa'a home in KwaMakutha. I continued to wonder how everybody could fit into my little Toyota Conquest, but Ncamisile tried to calm me down by suggesting that Phakamile and Wicky might have actually left already for KwaMakutha. Upon reaching Phakamile's house Ncamisile tricked me into the house by asking me to come and say hello to Phakamile's mother, but this trick backfired, for as soon as I alighted from the car leaving my keys in the ignition, Ncamisile locked my car, leaving my recording equipment stuck in the trunk. Upon entering the parlor of the house, people jumped up to their feet with the shout of "surprise!!!" These people had tricked me! How could they do that? I learned later that it was Nomusa and Phakamile's idea while the group had been deliberating on holding a farewell party to make it a surprise. On the dining table was a cake, of nearly 2 by 1 square feet, with the writing "We Love You Austin, Please Come Back to See Us." Unfortunately this occasion marked an important event that I participated in, but could not document. About an hour later, the PEPFAR film crew arrived. Among them were a White American woman, and a young White American man who seemed preoccupied with the fact that I was American, but did not speak English with an American accent. They were escorted by Nelli, another choir member. Mr. Freeth immediately asked about Austin, and quickly focused his camera on me. Apparently, they had told him about me and that they were organizing a farewell party for me.

The living room of Phakamile's home was becoming crammed now, so they decided to set up the cake, the drinks, and the food outside in the yard. There, the choir sang a few songs, including "Izizwe Mazihlome," "There Is No Other Name," and "Jehovah." Phumlani spoke first by thanking me for my time with them. Then he turned it over to any other member who wanted to say something, and everybody who spoke made it a point of duty to remind me that I must keep in touch and promise to come back to visit them. I was made to cut the cake, and I gave a short speech in response, including a few words of encouragement. The film crew interviewed me briefly on my experience with the group, after which they departed.

Sizwe and Xolani then drove me to Glenmore to pick up the spare key to my car while other choir members waited for us to return at about 6:30 pm. After a few moments of friendly interactions in the living room, the choir went into a meeting session. Phumlani spoke first, dropping a hint that there were a couple of invitations and important issues they needed to take care of. He wanted them to be brisk in deliberating on them with regard to who does what and how. Then he yielded the floor to Sizwe.

Sizwe started by explaining a few details about upcoming events and what he thought needed to be done about them. Then one member after another began to interject, often with more questions about things Sizwe had said, forcing him to explain further, and thereby also prompting others to voice an opinion. In a short while, the meeting was beginning to turn rowdy because there was so much arguing. Meanwhile, I was standing aside, wondering why this meeting was degenerating into bickering. I was worried that it was getting too late, some people's homes were far, and they needed to get to the city to catch the last buses to the townships particularly Inanda, KwaMashu, and KwaMukutha. I worried that Nokuthula, who was from Ngonyameni (a border town to Umlazi, but nevertheless a rural area), might actually find it difficult to get transportation home.

Suddenly, Sizwe's voice changed. He was standing in the center of the living room by the coffee table on which the remainder of my farewell cake had been placed, and was trying now to get everybody's attention. He began to say things that I did not understand. Then he went into some chanting; in response, the members sang the refrain Yea*!* Umhuu! 'Yes! Hawu! Amen!' By now, he had their attention, and their responses became like affirmations to his chants, which were two-to-three-word phrases. As the chanting went along, the pitch of his voice kept climbing, and so did the pitch of the group, as they responded to him. His voice sounded more and more strained, and I could see the arteries of his neck as he did the chanting. At some point, his voice reached a climactic pitch, whose sound he could no longer sustain; and it seemed this coincided with the end of the point he was trying to make, so he concluded by declaring, in an up-to-down vocal glide, that the message had been given "by the spirit" (*umoya oyincwele*), through him to them. To this, the choir responded by shouting *yiiiii!* in a high tone. The choir began to clap their hands, and started singing a song while dancing in a counterclockwise circle. After completing what seemed like a cycle of the chorus, another member leaped into the circle, and started another cycle of similar chant in a call-and-response format, concluding the cycle by declaring again that the word he had given was a message "from the spirit." The conclusion was again greeted with a similar exclamation, handclapping, and counterclockwise dance movement. Several other members took turns in voicing their opinions on the issues at stake in this rather "strange" meeting format.

As I watched and listened to this new call-and-response form of chanted speech interaction, it resembled more and more the style of prophecy and sermonic delivery among African independent churches, such as the Cherubim and Seraphim Church, and the Celestial Church of Christ in Nigeria. I asked Nokuthula what was going on, and she told me that they were actually imitating the Zionist Church. Nokuthula is a member of the Zulu Ibandla lamaNazaretha, but she is familiar with the practices of the Zionist Church. John Blacking, who studied this group of African independent churches in South Africa in the 1960s, described the social organization of their worship thus: "The order of services was supposed to be influenced by the Holy Spirit, who would bring the Word of God in the form of Bible texts, ideas for sermons, hymn themes, prophecies, and communal prayer" (1995: 209). According to him, "sermons were often interrupted by someone intoning a hymn, which was taken up by the congregation" (1995: 210). The interruptions were inspired by the idea expressed in the sermon or prophecy delivery, and the hymns served to strengthen the preacher spiritually to enhance his or her discourse. Blacking's study reveals a plan of worship that displayed freedom of musical expression and freedom-oriented eschatological theology. The organization of their worship therefore created a space for the negotiation of social processes wherein individuals found self-expression in the presence and with the help of others; and through participation in collective counterpoint, they achieved an experience they attributed to the Holy Spirit (1995: 209).

Later, Nomusa confirmed that they actually used the Zionist sermonic and prophecy delivery style every now and then during their meetings, especially if there was a sense that conflict might arise during the meeting. According to her, this had always proven useful by helping them reach resolutions on important issues without letting their discussions degenerate into bickering. What is interesting is how Siphithemba had managed to appropriate the Zionists' worship formulary as a mode of speech delivery in a rather non-worshipful context. It signaled to me that they were familiar with the modes of religious activities around them in their township communities, probably because they come from different denominational backgrounds. It was further evidence of their ability to adapt any available style of religious music and performance, so long as it helped them achieve desired goals, especially with regard to message transmission. Thus, in the face of HIV/AIDS, what is important is what works, and not necessarily what tradition or style one is following. In this meeting, the use of the Zionist sermonic and prophecy delivery style proved successful in preventing a heated argument, which I feared was on the verge of bruising feelings among members. It was also diagnostic of the sense of community especially as is contained in the *ubuntu* philosophy, an important aspect of which is the *indaba* (discussed in chapter 4), a meeting, consultative forum, or dialogue, a process in which competing or complementing parties engage to resolve or to prevent emergent crises in the community. What is unique in this instance however is that the choir's consultative forum became a musical *indaba.*

SUMMARY AND CONCLUSION

The music of the Siphithemba Choir as I have tried to demonstrate in this chapter is once again purposeful in their creative processes of song composition and performance. Although their song meanings had been addressed thematically in the preceding chapter, a close reading of musical processes and stylistics still reveals deeper meanings and significations. Their communal approach to song composition, the technics of layering multiple voices in a manner similar to Olly Wilson's theory of the "heterogeneous sound ideal" in African music, all point to the sense of community that define the organization of the choir as a HIV/AIDS support group and choral ensemble. In other words, the process of their musical production replicate in performance the same spirit that has guided their coming together from the very beginning at McCord Hospital.

Beyond the uniqueness of their story however, their process and stylistics of song and dance connect them further with the long tradition of Black choralism in South Africa, and African music in general. Hence even their dance and other bodily gestures are no longer merely designed for aesthetic purposes, than they are constructed with degrees of intentionality, imbuing them thus with deeper levels of meanings that continue to speak to their individual and collective experience of HIV and AIDS.

NOTES

1. The name substitution was occasioned by the interference of one of the scientists at the 2003 Conference in Boston, who went backstage to warn the choir against singing about God.
2. This song is one of the soundtracks that are heard in the musical *Ipi Ntombi* that premiered in 1974, but which gained notoriety after it was staged in Lagos during the 1977 Festival of African Arts and Culture (FESTAC). The musical was reproduced and recorded in the United States and Cape Town in the 1990s.

3. After arriving at the JFK Airport in New York, Mrs. Mhlongo was said to have been returned to Johannesburg by the U.S. immigration authorities because of problems associated with her visa.

4. This is taken from *American Zulu Mission: Extracts from the Journal Life and Light for Women,* courtesy of the Killi Campbell Africana Library, UKZN Durban. The date of the journal and identity of the writer of this passage are not evident in the document.

5. In IsiZulu, *ukuphatha* means "to touch, to feel." A dance style called *phatha phatha,* in which dance couples feel each other sensuously to music, grew out of *marabi* culture, a black urban pop culture of the 1930s through 1960s. In this instance, however, Siphithemba omits the coupling part of the dance, and incorporates the sensuous display of the hips.

Chapter 7

Dance without Drum

Playing the Politics of Culture in the Context of an Epidemic

On a night of July during my extended period of work with the Siphithemba Choir, a cocktail party was organized by McCord Hospital at the Zimbali Lodge at the Overport in Durban for Dr. Bruce Walker, the leading Harvard AIDs research scientist and his team. In line with what had become customary at the hospital, the Siphithemba Choir was asked to entertain the partiers. The event, which was broken up into three segments included a choral performance of favorite gospel tunes; buffet dining with wine; and another performance of several pieces that included gospel and traditional Zulu tunes. Whereas the first and second segments of the event took place on the veranda of the lodge, the third segment was moved into the hall because of poor lighting on the veranda, which impaired people's view of the choir's performance. During this third segment of the banquet, the choir sang different sets of gospel tunes, the choir's adaptation of "Nkosi Sikelel' iAfrika," "Sizwile Ukuthi," and "Isiyalo." The last was performed with a closing quotation from the traditional tune "Ikhalaphi."

The choir usually performed "Isiyalo" with a modern choreographed dance that incorporated elements of the *ukusina* foot-stamping, performed to a soundtrack accompaniment, but "Ikhalaphi" was performed purely as a traditional wedding song, integrated with the *ukusina* dance. In a rehearsal during the day at Umlazi, the choir made the decision not to use the instrumental soundtrack so they could make a smooth transition from *Isiyalo* to the second section of *Ikhalaphi.* In previous performances, the floor had been open to all choir members to demonstrate their facility with the dance, so they would all take turns coming to the front of the ensemble to demonstrate a solo dance. Sometimes, when performed exclusively to a Zulu audience, individual members of the audience would follow the trail of the choir to also demonstrate their facility with the dance, a practice that speaks to the communal nature of music making in African contexts, and the blurred boundaries between performers and audience (Nketia 1974: 21–34).

Something dramatic happened that night as soon as the choir made the transition from *Isiyalo* to *Ikhalaphi.* Some members of the choir, Nomusa and Zinhle rushed to the empty table that was by the wall in front of the audience and began vigorously pounding rhythmic patterns to accentuate the foot-stamping of the *ukusina* dance. The pounding of the beats on the table added energy to the dance. I thought, however, that the dance would have been more graceful if it had been accompanied with the *idlamu,* a large double-headed cylindrical drum (see figure 7.1). They had used the drum for their rehearsal during the day at Umlazi before the night's performance at the Zimbali Lodge. I had observed the dance style with the drum in several contexts: at regional and national choral festivals, at the Emmanuel Catholic Cathedral in Durban during the annual cultural mass, and among the male regimental ensemble of the Ibandla lamaNazaretha (the Zulu Nazarite Church). A certain commonality was persistent. Depending on the time signature of the song, the drummer subdivided the beats in the music and created a regular ostinato out of

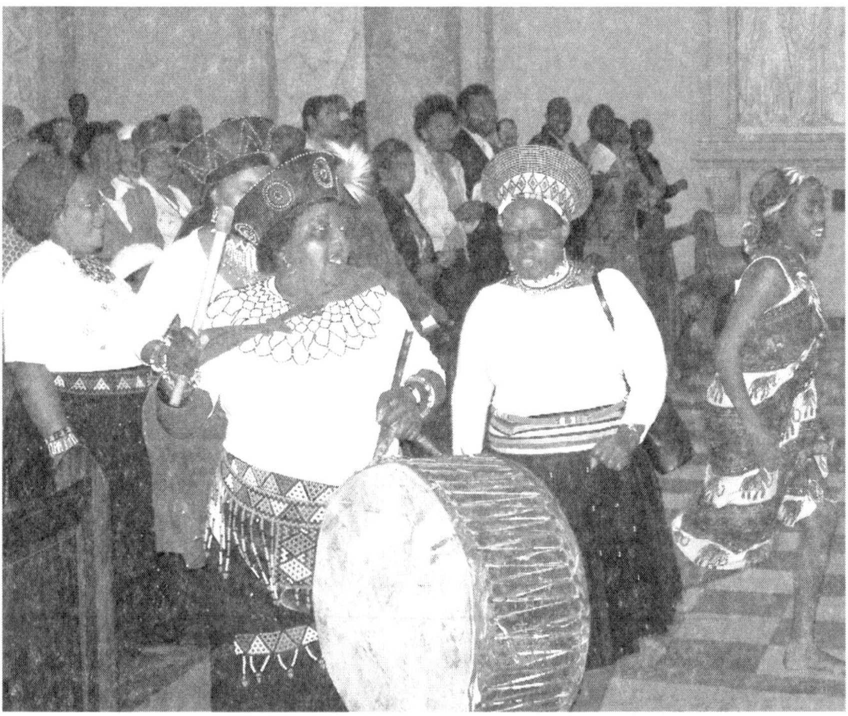

Figure 7.1 A Zulu woman playing *idlamu* during an entrance procession at a cultural mass at Emmanuel Catholic Cathedral, Durban.

the subdivisions in a subdued bass sound, but hammered a heavy, deafening beat to correspond with each stamp of the foot that the dancer demonstrated. Nomusa and Zinhle replicated this style of performance on the tabletop.

The event ended about midnight, and I drove Ncamisile and her two children and Xolani in my car to drop them off at Cato Crest and Umbilo, respectively, before returning to my room at the Glenmore Pastoral Center. On the way, I asked Xolani and Ncamisile about their decision to leave their drum behind at Umlazi and rather preferred to play on an empty table. Ncamisile responded, "there is no place for the drum *umfundisi*." I thought she simply meant that there was no space in the cars for transporting the drum to Zimbali Lodge. I accepted Ncamisile's explanation at the face value because Zinhle, who had directed the rehearsal at Umlazi during the day, had asked Wicky to bring out the *idlamu* drum to accompany the "Ikhalaphi" segment of the performance. In fact, at one point, they had asked me to play the drum for them so every member present could participate in the singing, as only a handful of them had been present at the rehearsal. By the end of the rehearsal, it appeared that the arrangement for a kombi bus that would transport the group to Zimbali Lodge had failed, so I packed my little Toyota Conquest with all the children and another adult member of the choir Nokuthula, while the bags of all the women filled the trunk of my car. Zinhle loaded the rest of the adults in the back of her "barky" (common South African parlance for pickup truck), with no room to spare. But, was it really the lack of space in the vehicles that was the reason? In fact, the drum could have fit into the trunk of my car, notwithstanding the women's bags. A revelation that explained their decision not to bring the drum was to be made later by Helga Holst, the medical superintendent of McCord Hospital.

THE DRUM CONTROVERSY

About a week following the event at the Zimbali Lodge I met with the medical superintendent in her office at McCord Hospital. During our meeting the superintendent recounted the history of the choir, placing it in the context of the story of the hospital as a church institution. She also shared her files with me, which contained photos of the choir's tours and performances, and cuttings of newspaper publications on the group and the hospital. I was getting ready to leave her office when she suddenly asked me about my faith, and what I thought about mixing elements and symbols of indigenous African religious practices with the Christian faith. Before I could respond, she went on to remark that I must know that superstition and the idea of the spirit is strong among the Zulu, and indeed among Africans. But she quickly added that the same is true among Europeans and people of European descent, more than is often acknowledged. I responded that, as one trained in theology, I am a strong believer in inculturation[1] and have no problems with letting peoples worship God in ways that are relevant to their own unique experiences and cultural ideals. Following my response she said, "Then ask them about their drum. . . . There was a controversy about it some time ago in this place. Ask them about it. If they trust you they will tell you something about it; then you should let me know."

I left the superintendent's office with so many questions running through my mind. What could the controversy have been? Why would she not tell me? Why had no one mentioned this so-called controversy to me, whether in the interview sessions or in informal conversations? Until now I had been made to believe that everything had been perfect for the choir in respect of their existence in and contributions to the hospital through their music and dance. In a later conversation, Phumlani Kunene, the choir director, explained that once during a trip to the United States with the superintendent, she had prevented them from bringing along the drum on the grounds that McCord is a Christian hospital and could not be associated with the use of the drum. Apparently she linked the drum with the ritual practices of Zulu traditional diviners (*izangoma*) and traditional healers (*izinyanga*), who used drums to invoke spirits or even to heighten their own spirit during ritual healing ceremonies. Phumlani explained however that the drum was also used traditionally for different purposes such as to signal the coming out of the king from the royal homestead and to transmit signals to the infantry regiments about an impending war. Its use in traditional Zulu dance is mainly to accompany and to accentuate the rhythm of the *ukusina* dance. According to him—and his explanation reflected the opinion of other members of the choir who later opened up to me about the drum controversy—the superintendent was mistaken in her interpretation of the spiritual significance of the drum. Some members believed that the superintendent's action amounted to an attack on their culture and identity as Zulu and Africans. It became clear to me from these conversations then that the choir's decision to not bring their drum to the event at Zimbali Lodge was a conscious effort to avoid a confrontation with the superintendent and not because of a lack of space in the vehicles providing transport to the event. The choir's performance that night at the Zimbali Lodge, their use of alternative accompaniment for the dance and the story behind the performance decision which unfolded later in the course of conversations with choir members and the medical superintendent of McCord Hospital raised the issue of cultural politics in a post-apartheid HIV/AIDS context. Examined against the background of the sociocultural and political history of South Africa, I argue that even in the context of a dare public health situation, the apartheid story still looms large, thus defining the nature of sociocultural relationships at the hospital made manifest in an AIDS-related music event. By setting the contestation over the use of the drum against the historical background of the colonial and apartheid cultural politics, I suggest that the controversy marked an instance of the continuation of the cultural politics that was integral to the apartheid system, which is now reproduced and replayed within the context of an HIV/AIDS music event. I interrogate what it means when the musical performance of HIV/AIDS becomes a space where the once opposing bodies in the system of apartheid engage in cultural contestation. Before proceeding however, I would like to examine further the drum in question and its place in Zulu musical culture.

THE *IDLAMU*, A ZULU MUSICAL INSTRUMENT

It is not clear how and when the *idlamu*, a double-headed cylindrical drum entered into and became a permanent feature of Zulu dance. The story of the controversy over the drum led me to investigate further the cultural use of the drum among some *izangoma.* In three different instances, the *zangoma* I spoke with insisted that the drums that are sold commonly in the market on Sydney Road in Durban are not their drums. Upon closer inquiry, I learned that the *zangoma* do not commonly purchase their drums from the open market; rather, they place a special order for them from specific makers, who appreciate the spirituality of the drum and its use in the cult. I observed *izangoma* dance music on a few occasions and ascertained that their dance formulary was different and devoid of the regimental-style *ngoma* music and the *ukusina* dance. Moreover, they used mostly other sets of drums called *izigubu* in Zulu. Hence, their performance style was different from that witnessed in *ngoma* music and *ukusina* dance. Some *izangoma* and drum makers on Sydney road with whom I spoke explained that *isigubu* (*pl. izigubu*) is a collective name for different shapes of drums. Some insisted that *idlamu* does not belong in that collective. A deeper inquiry into the history and meaning of the instrument revealed that *idlamu* was not originally a Zulu instrument. This assertion is premised on linguistic and comparative organological evidence that suggests *idlamu* is a corruption of the English word *drum*, as follows. The */i/* in *idlamu* is the subject prefix for noun class three, singular in IsiZulu. Since the phoneme /r/ does not exist in IsiZulu, Zulus tend to replace the /r/ sound in borrowed words with /l/.[2] Also, Zulu words, like those in most languages of sub-Saharan Africa, do not end with consonants. Thus the "shadow vowels" that are heard in the final consonants of English words are usually exaggerated to full vowel sounds, hence the /u/ in *idlamu* as a final vowel.

Further, the shape of the drum resembles in every respect the bass drum of the Western military regimental bands. The instrument probably entered Zulu musical culture by way of encounters with the British from the earliest days of the British military encampment at the port of Durban or possibly as late as the period of the First World War (see Kaemmer 2008: 403). Hence the Superintendent's attempt to proscribe the use of the drum may have been informed by erroneous assumptions about the place of the drum in Zulu culture.

Even if the *idlamu* did not have Western origins, the superintendent's action, notwithstanding her clear Christian intentions, could be construed as reminiscent of the colonial distortion of African cultural practices and condemnation of African values and worldviews as mere superstitions and savage idiosyncrasies (Etherington 2002: 422–39). Missionary efforts to suppress the music of African peoples, particularly those in Southern Africa, among whom they worked, have been well documented (Parrinder 1946: 190; Shaffer 1956: 39; Kaemer 1956: 57; Axelsson 1974: 91; Keteyi 1998: 23). Grant Olwage argues that the musical separations of race and ethnicity, as well as the institutional separations that occurred under apartheid, were rooted in the colonial and missionary ideologies of culture and identity politics (2008: 38–39). Fundamental to the European colonial and missionary engagement of African cultures, religions, and worldviews was the belief that they are primitive and evil (Etherington 2002: 422–39; Sindima 1992: 73–74; Turnbull 1962). For most early European missionaries, the civilization of Africans and ultimately their spiritual salvation lay in being wrested from their past and its "heathen" environment. Missionary suppression of African cultures was particularly evident in the area of music, a situation that in 1954 prompted Ghana's Philip Ghebo to challenge the missionaries against propagating "the idea that our music is primitive, fit only for the devil. I warn the missionaries to stop preaching that gospel, else there will be conflict between us and they will regret it in the end. They have done a lot to prohibit the music that is the center of our culture" (1954: 82). Ghebo's prediction of conflict on account of Europeans' attempt to prohibit African music came true in the case of the choir and McCord Hospital.

In South Africa, especially among the Zulu in the Natal region, the effort to extricate the African converts from their culture and indigenous ritual practices resulted in the establishment of mission stations including the Adams Mission in Amanzintoti by the American Congregationalists and the Marianhill Mission by the Roman Catholics where the *amakohlwa* (believers) were made to live apart from their original homesteads and kinsfolk. At these missions Africans were taught an idealized European lifestyle which was equated with Christian way of life; their degree of "civilization" was measured according to the degree they adopted the European lifestyle, even if superficially.

Apartheid was thus shaped by colonial missionary projects, which denigrated African cultures and in many instances proscribed many African cultural practices, particularly music. Once the missionary ideas about African and Zulu culture became entrenched they also became the basis for the formulation of the cultural components of the racial politics of the Union from the 1800s that culminated in the institutionalization of apartheid as State policy between 1948 and 1994. South African theologians, John and Steve de Gruchy (2005) lend credence to this historiography in their observation that apartheid, as it was practiced by the Afrikanner-led Nationalist Government, was first theologically conceived before it was given circular interpretation and political enactment. The proscriptive precedent that was set by the missionaries continued to influence the development of music in the mainstream mission churches. In the Roman Catholic Church the 1955 papal encyclical *Musicae Sacrae* and the Second Vatican Council constitution on the liturgy, which encouraged missionaries to promote local music for use in worship (Dargie 1997: 321), yielded little result.

From late 1970s and early 1980s however, following the efforts of David Dargie at the Lumko Missiological Institute in the Eastern Cape, marimba xylophones, inspired by the Zimbabwean marimba, developed at KwaNongoma music school in Bulawayo, began to be accepted as a church music instrument across Southern Africa (*ibid*, 322). Dargie, informed by his experience introducing marimba ensembles to Catholic congregations, reports that Africans' own non-readiness to embrace the use of local and indigenous musical forms and styles, as they were being pushed for by Lutheran missionary and musicologist Henry Weman for instance, and the utter rejection of the drum and drumming by the "educated elite" (1997: 231) constituted a stumbling block to African musical idioms and instruments gaining a pride of place in the mainstream churches. It is necessary to add, however, that the attitude of African elites was a result of the long-term cultural "(mis)education" that was perpetuated by the first generation of European missionaries beginning in the 1800s. It took the wave of political independence of several African states in the 1960s, which coincided with the Second Vatican Council (1962–65), and the emergence of African voices in the disciplines of philosophy and theology, especially the Kenyan Anglican priest and theologian, John S. Mbiti,[3] for African Christians to become open to indigenous African musical idioms. In South Africa, that coincided with the birth of the Black Consciousness Movement and the emergence of Black Theology. Yet, the call by Steve Biko, Barney Pityana, and pioneer exponents of South African Black Theology such as Bonganjalo Goba (1974: 65–73) and Gabriel Setloane (1973: 36–41) who, like Mbiti, looked back to "pre-colonial" African cosmologies and rituals as a basis for Africanizing the church, was overshadowed by the immediacy of the quest for political freedom. Moreover, their ideas were suspect in the eyes of State authorities, and also in the eyes of the still White-dominated church hierarchy.

Since 1990 however, the move to inculturate Christian worship and music in mainstream churches has gained traction.[4] However, this has been happening amid what are still largely segregated churches in South Africa. The implication is that majority of South Africans (Black and White alike) still do not have enough social and cultural interaction especially in religious spaces for attitudes to significantly change. White South Africans' experience of their surrounding African cultures is largely through the entertainment industry and the media, and vice versa. As Richard Dowden says, ". . . blacks and whites do not talk to, *nor do they know* each other. They live in their separate worlds with their very different thoughts and feelings about South Africa" (2009: 409). It is this persisting nature of the interracial relationships and the cultural attitudes that arise from it that can explain the misunderstanding that ensued between the superintendent and the Siphithemba Choir over the use of the *idlamu.* By seeking to prohibit the use of the drum, the superintendent triggered memories of apartheid under which system the politics of culture and the cultural domination of Africans by Europeans comprised ideological bedrock (Comaroff and Comaroff 1985: 1–22). According to South African Jesuit theologian Xolile Keteyi, "Black people have used music . . . to tell the story of their trauma and pain; to proclaim their aspirations and affirm their humanity" (1998: 28). Again some choir members I interviewed construed the superintendent's action as an attack on their culture and identity as Africans and Zulu. From my conversations with them, and Keteyi's words above, one could argue that, as a group of young men and women whose lives have been severely impacted by the burdens of the HIV/AIDS and social stigma, the superintendent's actions constituted a double attack on their aspirations and the affirmation of their humanity their participation in the choir was meant to afford. According to Phumlani, events similar to this forced them to shift their perspective about their struggle with HIV and AIDS. Born out of a consciousness of their mutual struggle with HIV/AIDS, a disease that has been so politicized, they now construe themselves as engaged in the struggle first as individuals, second as a group with shared experiences, and third as African people who must raise their voices for the African cause in the context of the global AIDS pandemic.

On another level, although their music may function as a culturally based form of intervention in the HIV/AIDS problem, the musical performances sometimes also reveal other underlying political dynamics that expose what some scholars of post-apartheid studies have characterized as the residues of apartheid-era sentiments, which "continue to influence, shape and limit the trajectory of development of a post-apartheid order for the foreseeable future" (Norval 1996: 1; see also Fassin 2007: 72). The controversy over the use of the *idlamu* drum by the Siphithemba Choir and how that has impacted their musical choices is particularly illustrative of this reality. While in other cases traditional practices and cultural symbols have been mobilized as a means of securing legitimacy in grassroots education (McNeil 2011), at McCord Hospital the *idlamu* as a musical instrument was excluded from performance by ascribing meaning to it that challenged its legitimate place within the space of a Christian health service.

Also, the controversy over the use of the drum raised the question about how and why the context of the fight against HIV and AIDS became once again the space for contestation over cultural symbol and meaning. During my meeting with the superintendent Helga Holst, I asked to visit the hospital chapel, but she disclosed that there was none. Sensing my astonishment she declared "the entire hospital is a sanctuary." This declaration showed a strong and extant belief by the White-dominated management of the hospital that the health institution is primarily a spiritual space. For her—and probably for some, or perhaps even most, White people in management—what is spiritually Christian is incompatible with, and cannot contain any, African-derived cultural elements. In contrast, my interactions with the choir show that the choir members see themselves as a Christian music ensemble. Though they belong to different Christian denominations, according to Phumlani, Xolani, and Wicky, they made a conscious decision to stick to the performance of gospel music, with little tincture of Zulu traditional tunes. According to Xolani, "Singing made me realize that I could serve God anywhere." It is for this reason that they told me that they in fact prefer to be designated as "Siphithemba Gospel Choir." Though they are all HIV-positive, they prefer to be described as preaching the gospel of hope in the face of HIV/AIDS. They prefer this designation to the more common tendency to refer to them as the "HIV Choir." They see themselves as a Christian group, but they do not shy away from adopting cultural elements that they regard as an integral part of their African identity, a sign of growing awareness among "Black South Africans that Christianity did not require complete Europeanization; one might convert to Biblical Christianity without losing one's cultural identity" (Muller 2004: 196). And, one way in which Black South Africans, and indeed the Zulu, have strived to retain their cultural identity is through their music. Like I discussed in chapter 5, the Siphithemba Choir does not see any inherent contradictions between the African cultural idioms they use in their performances, their Christian faith, and the gospel message they purport to preach. Xolani made the point that they "preach the gospel and give hope through [their] music." Asked how he sees the consistency of incorporating traditional songs with "preaching the gospel," he responded, "Because they are part of who we are as African people, I think it is okay, we can still praise God with traditional music, because we are doing good work with it." Thus for Xolani, and for the choir members, the appropriateness of their use of traditional music and the *idlamu* consists in the "good work" that they do with their music as opposed to the "spiritual meanings" they might hold in the traditional setting.

SUMMARY AND CONCLUSION

My aim in this chapter has been to use this case study of a music event in a HIV/AIDS context to examine the issue of the politics of culture as it relates to the use or non-use of the *idlamu* as a musical instrument by the Siphithemba Choir. By examining the issue raised by use of the *idlamu* against the background of apartheid as cultural policy and the history of colonialism and Christian missionization in South Africa, questions are raised about the implications of the contestations over the drum as an artifact that is imbued with cultural symbolism and meaning. I suggest that the drum controversy at McCord Hospital, which informed the performance choices of the Siphithemba Choir has implications in post-apartheid discourse. One is forced to ask the question, what is "post" in "post-apartheid"? In other words, what does it mean to speak about post-apartheid considering the case of this HIV/AIDS-related music event and the drum controversy?

Since the democratic transition in 1994, "post-apartheid" as a discourse has preoccupied scholars (Freund and Padayachee 1998: 16–22; Wilson 2000: 75–98; Ramphele 2001: 1–17), who analyze the prospects for future development against the background of the legacies of apartheid. While the discourse has focused largely on issues related to politics and economic development, the cultural conditions of apartheid are yet to be completely undone and have scarcely been addressed as relevant panacea for sustainable human and socioeconomic development. "Post-apartheid" presupposes the cessation of the conditions that defined apartheid. It is a forward-looking analysis of the legacies of apartheid in which scholars tend to make projections about the prospects for future development as those conditions and legacies recede into memory. In this regard, post-apartheid as a discourse, as mentioned above, has largely focused on issues of politics and economic development plus the conditions of human rights in South Africa. The discourse has seldom paid attention to religion and culture, which were the major cornerstones of the initial formulation of apartheid policy. Not even the Truth and Reconciliation Commission (TRC) addressed the issue of cultural violations that were visited upon Africans, on their psyche and sacred places, by the Apartheid State and the mission churches. During one of my research trips to South Africa, I visited the *Isivivani*—Freedom Park in Pretoria of which the original intent in the construction was to address some of the cultural violations of Africans and the Khoi and San peoples and other inhabitants of South Africa (see www.freedompark.co.za/). In a conversation however with Manshilo

Motsei, South African feminist writer and cultural activist, she disclosed that the Park only serves as a memorial and its conceptualization did not include an effort at reconciling and resolving the cultural violations that the history of apartheid and the colonialism brought upon the inhabitants of the land. The implication is that, not only are aspects of the cultural legacies of apartheid still in place, but in fact the cultural conditions and sentiments that characterized apartheid are still strong in many places, as seen in the instance of the *idlamu* controversy at the McCord Hospital.

When therefore in 1996 then president Mandela declared HIV/AIDS "the next struggle," an invocation of the antiapartheid struggle, I suggested he triggered a symbolic linking of apartheid with the current experience of HIV and AIDS. Mandela's idea of "the next struggle" may have been about the public health situation; yet, several years after his declaration, a community experience and collective (albeit interracial) fight against HIV/AIDS was the context where the once opposing bodies in the system of apartheid engaged in cultural contestation, with music—use of a Zulu instrument—at the center of that struggle. This situation illustrates, as it were, Grant Olwage's suggestion that the "end of apartheid may not be construed as the end of the apartheid story" (2008: 8). Again, and finally, the music event under consideration here is AIDS-related, but it is also diagnostic of the fact that while music comprised part of apartheid's logic of separations as well as helped to take it apart, as Olwage argues (see also Byerly 1998: 1–44); the space for highlighting some of the "non-conclusions and continuations" of aspects of the apartheid story is found in this AIDS music event, even when the major actors in the contestations of meaning have clear and honest intentions.

NOTES

1. I use "inculturation" here as a term that is employed in theological circles in reference to the adaptation of Christian teachings and practices to local cultures, and how the cultures shape the evolution of Christian practices. It differs from the anthropological term "enculturation" which denotes the process of cultural formation of an individual.
2. Because of the absence of /r/ in isiZulu, many Zulu who are not very proficient in English would pronounce the Rand, the South African currency, as *"ilandi,"* replacing the /r/ with /l/ while adding /i/ at the beginning as part of noun class three subject prefix, and a final /i/ as an exaggerated shadow vowel.
3. See, for example, Mbiti (1969), *African Religions and Philosophy.*
4. Between 2005 and 2007 I documented series of experimentations in this direction at the Emmanuel Catholic Cathedral in Durban in the form of the cultural mass, and in the Methodist Church in Durban.

Chapter 8

The Siphithemba in Politics of Identity and Representation

In the introductory chapter, I highlighted how during my first encounter with the Siphithemba Choir, their songs and style of performance got me wondering in the first place about the insertion of racial ideas into their songs. As my work with the group progressed, I documented several of their songs a closer examination of which revealed multiple references to Africa and Blackness. Some of the songs include "Siyaphela IsiZwe seNkosi" (The nation of the Lord is finishing), "Siyakubonga Somandla" (We thank you Almighty), and "Jehova." In these songs, "Africa" is conflated with the "Black Race" (*abantu abamnyama)*, or "Black Nation" (*Umnyama yezwe*) in a manner that is similar to what Anthony Appiah has discussed as a notion of Africa that is defined not by geography, but rather by demarcation along the lines of skin color (1992: 3–27). By so doing they thus signal a global ethnic/racial consciousness in the context of the HIV/AIDS discourse. The choir conductor, Phumlani Kunene, and other members explained that the referencing of Black or Africa in their songs is premised on their understanding of Africans and people of African descent as comprising the majority of the victims of the AIDS pandemic. Scholarships on public health that discuss the racial disparities in the HIV/AIDS prevalence (Prejean et alia 2011; Adimora and Shoenback, 2002: 707–712; Krieger, 2003: 1655–1671; Okigbo et al., 2002: 615–653; Quinn, 1993: 305–320[1]) bring validity to this observation, one that is implied in the question that Xolani Zulu posed to me thus, "Why umfundisi [father]; why is it that everywhere you go, even in America, it is always the Black people that are suffering from this [HIV/AIDS] problem?"

In this chapter I explore two issues, namely the issue of race and African identity and the politics of representation as they are articulated in Siphithemba songs. I examine the ways in which the Choir through their music have participated in these levels of politics in local and international contexts by drawing from and examining specific moments, actions, and materials that define the dynamics. I suggest that the Choir's articulations of the sense of race in their songs are not by chance, but rather based on conscious compositional and performative choices that are informed by their perceptions of the sociopolitical and economic inequities that have shaped the local and global HIV/AIDS discourse. Under the politics of representation, I argue that the choir consciously engages in the process of offering a counter-narrative to the AIDS discourse as it pertains to Africa using the circumstances of their relationship with the scientists involved in medical science research on AIDS. Secondly, the choir uses their contextual encounters with American audiences to highlight aspects of the AIDS experience in the West, which scarcely form part of the larger conversation on the global AIDS experience, but which has tended to paint the disease in a one-sided light as solely an African (and developing-world) problem.

ISSUES INFORMING BLACK IDENTITY EXPRESSIONS IN SIPHITHEMBA SONGS

Siphithemba's race consciousness in the context of the HIV/AIDS experience is informed by more than the statistical evidence of Blacks as comprising the majority of the victims of the disease. I suggest rather that their consciousness has been shaped by the function of several related factors: the nature of the human immuno deficiency virus itself,[2] the global politics of AIDS, the lingering effects of apartheid, and the continuing interracial acrimony in a post-apartheid environment. I argue therefore, that these factors have impacted how the HIV/AIDS pandemic is perceived and interpreted through the lens of race in South Africa, thereby generating a specific set of socio-cultural production. Hence the Siphithemba Choir uses its music to perform Black South African experience, and to negotiate a sense of Black and African identity within the context of the AIDS discourse.

First, the apartheid history left lingering effects in virtually all sectors of life in present-day South Africa (*see* Karim et al., 2009: 921; Covadia et al., 2009:60951). The current public health challenges are at least partly rooted in the historical legacies of apartheid. With regard to HIV/AIDS, scholars of public health and social medicine (Brummer, 2002: 1–26; Joechelson et al., 1991: 157–173; Seftel, 1988: 17–22) identify the labor migrant system under apartheid, with its associated overcrowded male hostels and squatter settlements, and deliberately underdeveloped health services for Blacks as what "provided a favorable environment for efficient transmission of HIV" (Karim et al., 2009: 921).

In addition to the structural factors, self-contradictory social attitudes shaped the apartheid government's policy on AIDS from the beginning. For example, the belief that HIV was a predominantly White homosexual problem informed the Department of National Health and Population Development establishment of AIDS-training, information, and counseling centers only in major White urban areas beginning in 1988 (Nattrass, 2007: 38). At the same time, the apartheid government labeled AIDS a "black disease" just to reinforce racial prejudices about Black sexual promiscuity (Karim, 2009: 923). Thus racial profiling was a significant aspect of the government's initial response to HIV. All Black people were prevented from donating blood, while HIV-positive migrant miners from Malawi, Mozambique, and other neighboring countries were deported (Nattrass 2007: 38).

The government's labeling AIDS as "black disease" was a cause for curiosity among Black South Africans, especially because HIV was first reported in South Africa among White homosexuals in 1982 (*see* Karim et al., 2009: 922). Nearly five years after the first appearance of the virus in the Republic, no singular seroprevalence survey conducted among pregnant women and hospital patients including in the Black community identified any infected individual (Karim and Karim, 1992: 484). By 1988 however, the heterosexually transmitted subtype C was first reported in the general population and the Black community, and between 1990 and 1994 the infection rate doubled in the Black community on a yearly basis. Also allegations were made—albeit with inconclusive investigation—at the Truth and Reconciliation Commission (TRC) in 1998 concerning the storing and possible dissemination of HIV-infected blood in the Black community as part of bio-weaponry project by the South African defense ministry.[3] Unfortunately the non-conclusion of the investigation left room for the allegation to transform into imagined reality. I had a conversation with a Black student at the Nelson Mandela Medical School during one of my research trips to South Africa. Referencing the allegations that were made at the TRC, the student insisted that the apartheid government intentionally introduced HIV in the Black community. Like this young medical student, members of the Siphithemba Choir and ordinary South Africans tend to reference the "revelations" at the TRC as evidence that the apartheid government spread HIV in the Black community.

The nature and timeline of the appearance of the virus in various communities in South Africa, and the TRC hearings on bio-weaponry thus account partly for the suspicion about intentional introduction of HIV into the Black community by the apartheid government. The suspicion was, and still remains strong even among politicians[4] prompting the Rhodes University social anthropologist Virginia van der Vliet to critique the accusations being labeled against the White-controlled National Party as instigating among White voters that AIDS would reduce the Black majority to a minority population in a period of five years (2004: 48–96). These conversations on HIV/AIDS have serious affect on the AIDS discourse in South Africa, so that the polemics surrounding the public debate on AIDS according to Didier Fassin, "are ever more influenced by racialist readings . . . in ways that are ever more radical" (2007: 72).

The "conspiracy theory" concerning the intentional and strategic introduction and dissemination of HIV in the Black South African community by the White apartheid government started gaining momentum once again during my extended research stay in South Africa in 2007, when it was announced that the microbecides gel that was being tested in KwaZulu-Natal (primarily among Black women) had failed, and in fact had proven to increase the risk of infection. Meanwhile the insistence of the White scientist and professor at the University of Cape Town who was overseeing the research project to continue with the testing of the gel in South Africa drew outrage from the Black community.

On their part, the Siphithemba Choir experienced issues at the McCord Hospital that also forced them to analyze their experience of the HIV/AIDS in terms of race. For example, McCord Hospital had two support groups, one for Blacks and another for Whites and Coloreds. A member of the hospital management explained to me that the separation was made to accommodate the Whites and Coloreds, the majority of whom were employed and could not meet on Tuesdays with the Black patients. The separation of the two groups nevertheless reminded members of the Siphithemba Choir of the separation of the racial groups under apartheid. Gugu *(pseudonym)* commented on this thus, "many of us were getting sick and some were dying, but we see them [*White patients*], they say that they are also positive, but they looked better. I think because they have jobs and making money, but for us, we have nothing."

Also, the controversy over the *idlamu,* which I addressed in the preceding chapter recalled for members of the Siphithemba Choir the cultural politics that was at the core of (South) Africa's political history. Like I stated, some choir members believed that the superintendent's prohibition of the drum amounted to an attack on their culture as Africans, especially because their music is used to "tell the story of their trauma and pain; to proclaim their aspirations and affirm their humanity" (Keteyi 1998: 28). The prohibition of the drum by the superintendent therefore turned the context of the fight against HIV/AIDS into a space for contestation over cultural symbol and meaning, thereby triggering memories of apartheid under which system the politics of culture, and the cultural domination of Africans by Europeans comprised an ideological bedrock.

On another level, the legal battle between the South African government and thirty-nine international pharmaceutical companies over the importation and/or manufacture of cheaper generic antiretroviral drugs had impact on the public discourse on HIV and AIDS in South Africa. In addition to the argument for patent rights, there were loud speculations about whether Africans could satisfactorily handle the complexity of the ARV regimen. The fact that African countries, including South Africa, Uganda and Kenya had been major centers for the clinical trial of anti-AIDS drugs seemed to be inconsequential in the debate. During a performance at the conference in Boston, Zinhle Thabethe who gave the keynote speech in place of Mrs. Mhlongo used the medium of the concert stage to thank the gathering of scientists for their good work in developing the anti-AIDS drugs. At the same time, she spoke out against those who made the arguments that "Africans are incapable of handling the antiretroviral regimen" as a reason for delaying the delivery of the drugs to Africa (*see* Hainsworth 2006). In this speech, Zinhle argued that she is a living example of the success of ARV in an African environment.

The complex interplay of the socio political and cultural factors thus shaped Siphithemba Choir's use of choral singing to perform their African and Black identity. It was for this reason that the choir conductor Phumlani Kunene made the striking Pan-Africanist/Pan-Black comment about their music when he stated, "we are aware of these issues, and so whenever we are singing, . . . we believe that we are talking not just about ourselves, but for Africa and for Black people everywhere." Phumlani's statement echoes what ethnomusicologist Thomas Turino (2000: 7–8) noted as shared cross-cultural sensibility of nationalist minds with members of similar class and sociopolitical and racial or ethnic background across national boundaries. Hence to the Siphithemba Choir, they share common background and experience with all people of African descent around the world who appear to be the majority of the victims of HIV and AIDS in most national territories where they live. The consciousness articulated by Phumlani and which is evidenced in Xolani's rather rhetorical question thus clearly undergirds the textual mainstay of some of the choir's songs and the nature of their musical stylistics in general.

MUSICAL EXPRESSIONS OF AFRICANNESS

Siphithemba Choir's performance of African and Black identity is realized through the textual mainstay of their songs, the integration of song and dance, and the use of indigenous Zulu-derived concert dress to reflect an African worldview and aesthetics.

Three of their songs that most clearly speak about African and Black experience of HIV/AIDS have been listed above. Siyakubonga Somandla is an adaptation of a pre-existing song "Yihla Umoya oyiNcwele, Usindisi Afrika"

(May the Holy Spirit descend, and Africa will be saved), which the choir begins by singing about "hope" as a way to put their signature on the song. Upon completing the first part of the song that speaks about hope, followed by repeated humming of the melody, the choir returns to the original text, only now performed in English and with a shift into a grammatical genrundive of obligation in contrast to the pleading nature of the original version.

Original version

Yehla Moya oyiNgcwele
Usindise i-Afrika
May the Holy Spirit descend
And Africa will be saved

Siphithemba version

Siyakubonga Somandla
Usinikile ithemba
We thank you Lord
Because you gave us hope

The Holy Spirit must come down
And Africa must be saved.

The composer of the original version of the song is unknown. Archival sources however show that the song features frequently in the annual Good Friday Ecumenical Services that are organized by the Diakonia Council of Churches in Durban. In fact my review of the program of service from 1998 through 2014 revealed continued appearance of the song the entire sixteen years. The Good Friday Ecumenical Service, the first of which took place in 1978 is part of what was known as *protest liturgy* that were organized by Churches in defiance of the Apartheid State. The very first service was to protest against the State for detaining several members of the clergy who led a rally against Bantu Education.[5] Diakonia continues to organize this service yearly as a way to engage the masses with the present social, economic, and political challenges in post-apartheid South Africa. Featuring the song every year in the ecumenical service shows it's close association with the liturgical event. The Siphithemba Choir was the host choir for the 1998 service whose theme was "Ukuphila Ngegazi Lika Jesu" (Life through the Blood of Jesus). It was in fact at this ecumenical service that the choir adapted the song the first time, thus inserting their "hope" signature into the song. Now performed in the context of HIV/AIDS, the song speaks about salvation for Africa, representing a vision and consciousness about the African experience of HIV/AIDS.

Furthermore, I was curious about the choir's shift in mood, namely the use of the gerundive in their version of the song. I pointed out to them the difference between their version and the version that appeared in several editions of the Good Friday service program. To this Nomusa Mpanza responded,

> You know this problem [HIV/AIDS] is too much. Even for us it is too much. So sometimes, people want to give up hope. But for us we have hope. We don't give up, because we know that we are not going to die, all of us, no matter what anybody thinks.

Thus for Nomusa, and for the choir members, the use of the gerundive is an expression of their resilience, confidence, and faith in God as one who has the power to turn the tide of the AIDS epidemic in their community and in Africa in general.

I already examined "Jehovah," and "Siyaphela IsiZwe seNkosi" more extensively in chapter 6. I reintroduce them briefly in this place however in order to examine them further to the extent that they speak directly about African and Black experience of AIDS.

Jehovah (Excerpt)

Jehovah, Jehovah
Qhawe elinkhulu ngonyama yezwe

Sikhala kuwe
Sinxusa kuwe
Siphe amandla
Sinqoba izilingo

Jehovah, Jehovah *Jehovah, Jehova*
Great hero of the Black nation
We cry to you
We plead you
Give us power
To conquer temptations

The song opens with a theme that speaks of back nationalism, by referring to God as "the great hero of the black nation." It is both a plea for God's intervention as well as a verbal act of prostration before God as the omnipotent who alone can salvage the situation by helping the nation to conquer the disease.

"Siyaphela IsiZwe seNkosi" speaks to the issue of Black and African identity succinctly too. Lyrically, the first section of the song addresses the community directly, but the community is more than local: it is Africa.

Like I observed at the beginning of this chapter, there is the understanding that Africans are the majority of the victims of the disease, but also there is the perceived notion that an international, albeit Western corporate conspiracy was making Africans' access to the antiretroviral regimen difficult. These factors forced the choir to construe themselves as raising their voices on behalf of Africa as much as for themselves and their local KwaZulu-Natal community. It is in the light of this understanding that Phumlani, echoing other choir members who commented on whether the use of the word *Africa*[6] is racially conceived, commented on their awareness of "these issues," namely the perceived global politics of AIDS, such that they devote and dedicate their music to the course of the African and Black world experience of AIDS.

The sense of community in this song is evident on two levels: on the first level, articulated in the a segment, Africa is referred to as the "nation of the Lord," and according to Phumlani, this reference links the current problem with the historical experience of Africans and Black people as victims of the world's problems. The song then goes on to call on Africans to "rise up and fight"—a recognition that only Africans are in the best position to understand and solve their own problems. It emphasizes the need to join hands in combating the disease.

The Black-nationalist undertone in the song reflects the singers' commitment to use of music on behalf of Africa, the center of the global AIDS pandemic. By referring to their community—whether as a choir, a local Zulu community, Africa, and Black people—as God's people or "nation of the Lord," Siphithemba reiterates its commitment to a relationship with God, in whom they repose their faith and hope.

On another level, the song is educational, as observed in rallying calls to the community to "rise up and fight." As a group, the choir is engaged in the mission of bringing the message of hope to its people; but it also engages in the work of educating and mobilizing the community in the fight against HIV/AIDS. Finally, by representing the response to HIV/AIDS as a form of struggle, the song recalls former president Nelson Mandela's characterization of HIV/AIDS in South Africa as "the next struggle." The choir members thus successfully inscribe themselves in the South African tradition of deploying choral music in their struggles. In this way, they comprise a new voice in an old tradition. In effect, the significance of this song, in addition to being a favorite of the choir, is that it embodies the character of the choir as a faith community. Their other songs each reflect some aspects of who they are as a faith group engaged in the struggle with HIV/AIDS, but "Siyaphela Isizwe SeNkosi" captures this character in its entirety.

Furthermore, and in considering the three songs together on a broader level, I had wanted to know how the choir members would respond to a situation where their audience construed their constant referencing of Africa and the "Black Race" as "the nation of the Lord" as excluding other nations from God's fold.

Phumlani and Xolani responded, "We are all children of God." One evening after completing a recording rehearsal at Umlazi, and while driving with him back to Umbilo, I pressed Xolani further on the issue, and he responded thus:

> You know *umfundisi*,[7] God is not the God of any particular people. He is the God of Black people too. We are his children, so he is supposed to protect us like he is protecting other people. So we are not saying that only Africa belongs to God: instead, we are saying that we are also his people.

The reference to Africa in the songs, and the lumping of the entire "black race" into one "nation," is symbolic. Their equating Black people with Africa recalls Kwame Anthony Appiah's discourse as indicated earlier on the invention of an Africa that is more than a geographical entity, but one defined and demarcated along the lines of skin color (1992: 3–27, 62).

In regard to calling Africa "the nation of the Lord," it is not uncommon in a society where theology has shaped the racially violent politics of the past, for specific ethnic or racial groups to consciously or unconsciously lay claim to a special relationship with God. Afrikaner nationalism for instance, as has been argued by South African theologians John and Steve de Gruchy (2005), was forged on the assumption of being a chosen race, wherein the movement of the vortrekkers in search of a "homeland" became a typology that reenacted the biblical exodus. Similarly (as shown in chapter 5), Isaiah Shembe, founder of the Zulu Ibandla lamaNazaretha, sought to counteract the White claim to superiority and a "special relationship with God" by drawing upon biblical imageries to interpret the Zulu experience of oppression under the colonial and settler government in Natal. On the part of the Siphithemba Choir, "Siyaphela Isizwe" is evidence of influence by the racially charged political history of South Africa. Hence the racial polarization that plays out in the HIV/AIDS discourse finds expression in the ensemble's music. Therefore, by ascribing an ecclesial status to this constantly shifting and expanding community, the geographical and theological are conflated.

While the three songs that I have discussed so far are largely religious music, the choir conductor Phumlani and another member Nomusa revealed that they also incorporate traditional Zulu songs because of their amenability to integration with dance. According to Phumlani, "these traditional songs have a way of making people want to dance." As a result, the *ukusina*, an indigenous Zulu dance that is characterized by energetic high kick and heavy stamping of feet is the preferred dance style. Most importantly, dance is a way to project their distinctive African identity in performance particularly at international concerts. Traditional songs paired with dance also comprise part of the appropriate medium of speaking to their South African audience in recognizable form.

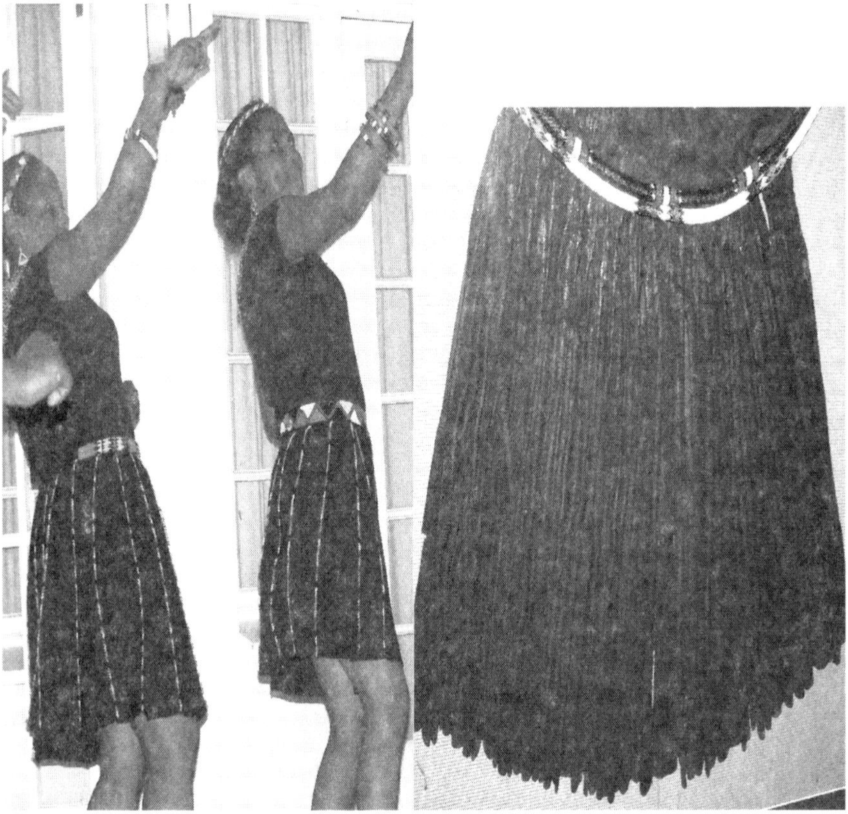

Figure 8.1 Illustrations of the similarity between the traditional Zulu *isidwaba* and the Siphithemba skirts.

The need to connect with local audiences and project an African identity also informed the choir's use of traditional Zulu dresses as part of their performance regalia. Although the choir had several different uniforms while still at McCord Hospital, they have retained just three. One is a black skirt decorated with Zulu bead embroidery along the pleats for the women. According to Mrs. Mhlongo, the skirt was modeled after the *isidwaba,* a traditional skirt, made from cowhide that is died black. The choir women wear the skirt with a black waistband of Zulu beads, a black top, and an embroidered-style Zulu necklace. Sometimes the women cap their regalia with headbands made of beads, or with *isicholo* (pl. *izicholo*) (figure 8.1), a crown that is traditionally sown from twigs or fiber worn by married women. Whereas *isicholo* is traditionally married women's attire in Zulu society, these days the hat stands as one of the cultural symbols of the Zulu nation, and is therefore ubiquitous in the tourist markets in South Africa. Hence the women of the Siphithemba

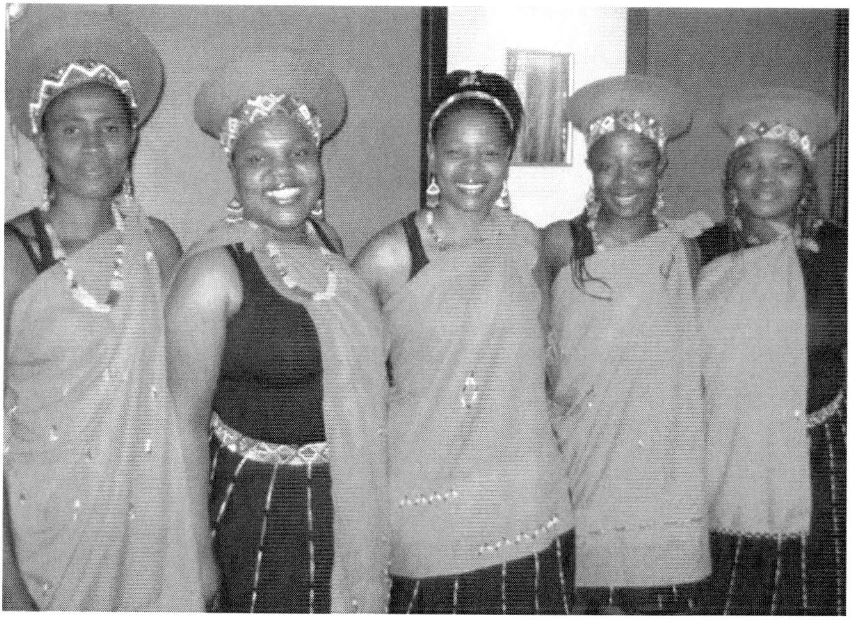

Figure 8.2 Some female Siphithemba Choir members pose in full regalia.

Choir wear the hat, not as married women (though some of them are married), but as a way to project Zulu cultural identity. At other times, the women add an *ibhayi* (figure 8.2) over their shoulders.

The men's attire, designed by Xolani at his African Vision Shop, is modeled after those worn by Zulu *maskanda* artists (figure 8.3). The pants and a petit-coat top display a multicolor quilted design, and the headgear is an animal skin headband. All components of the uniforms are colors of the South African national flag—which exemplifies the republic as a "rainbow nation."

Another uniform worn by the choir is a green superwax print[8] with the title "African American Heritage" and images of African leaders, including Emperor Haile Selassie, and African American leaders, including Dr. Martin Luther King, Jr., and Marcus Garvey (figure 8.4). These clothes were given to the choir by a South African Zulu family that lived in Los Angeles when the choir toured the United States in 2003. According to Phumlani, "We did not buy the clothes; a brother gave it to us in America. But we liked it so much, it says something about black people."

Victor Turner (1980: 12) described the human body surface as "the symbolic stage upon which the drama of socialization is enacted." Fashion, albeit what people wear, and the ways in which the body surface is adorned thus comprise part of that socialization, that is, a process of self-enactment as a

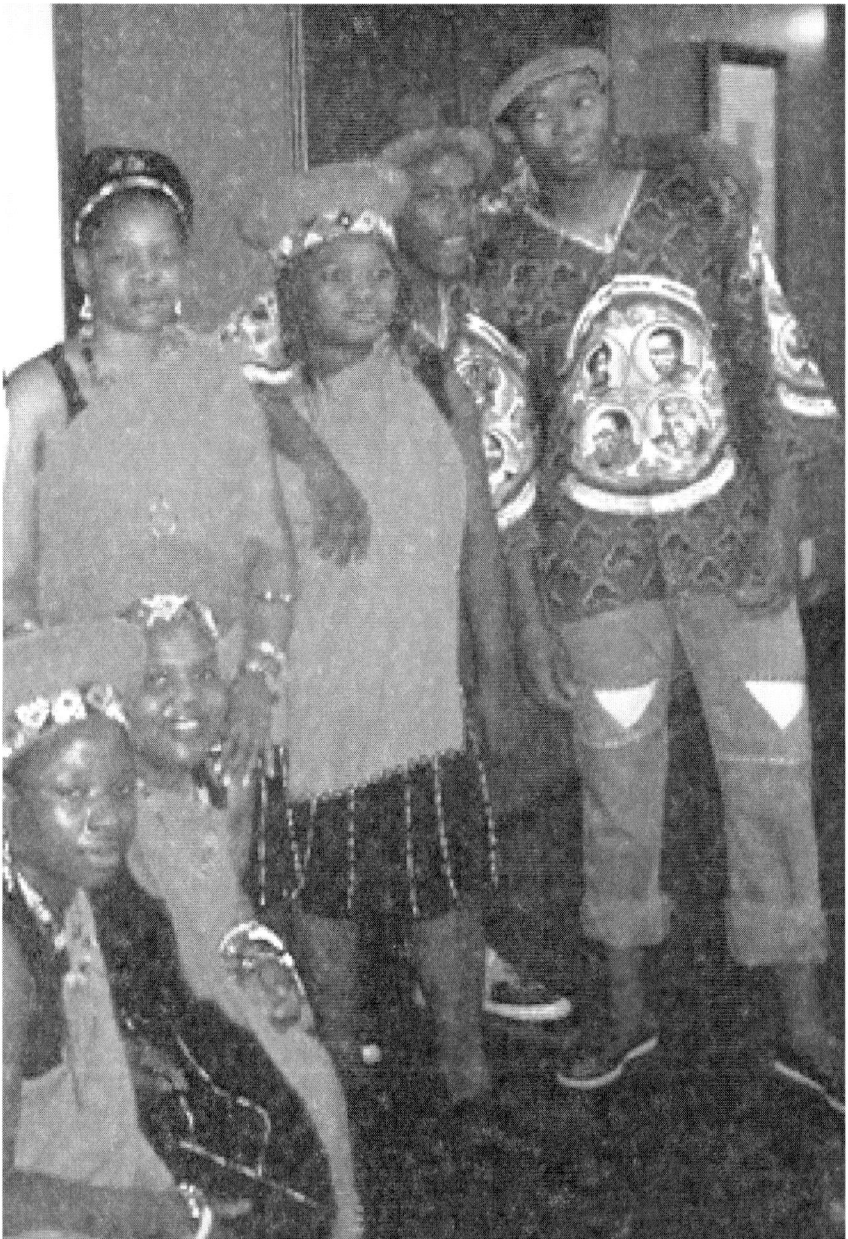

Figure 8.3 Some men and women of the Siphithemba Choir.

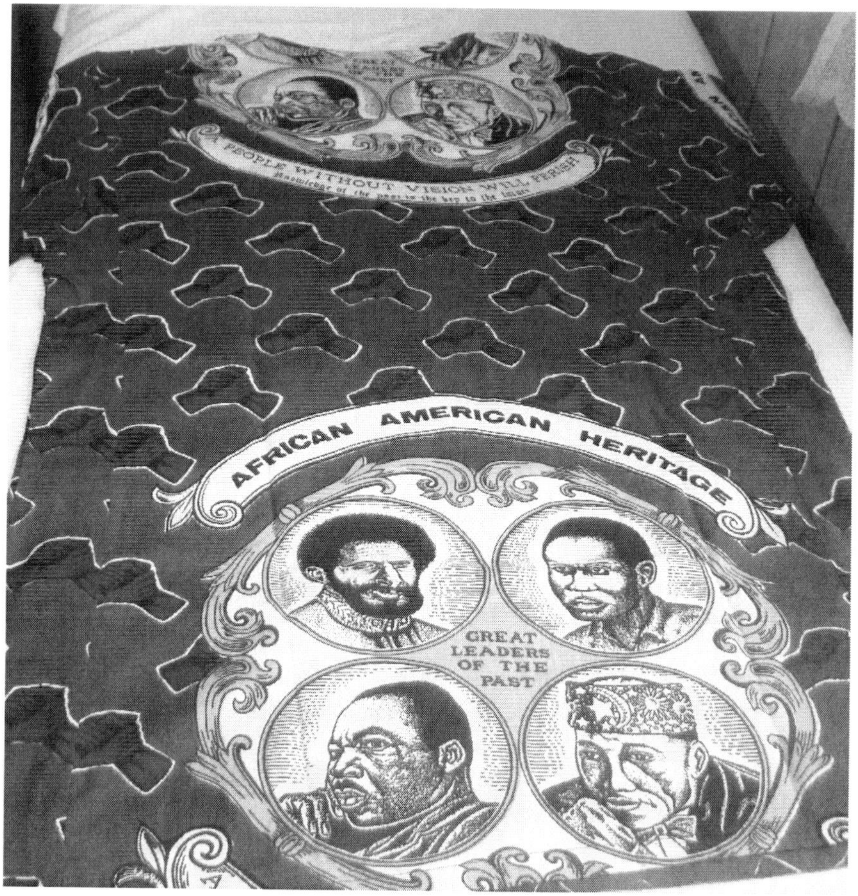

Figure 8.4 A front view of the African American print shirt.

member or members of specific culture group. It is the process "for constituting the social self, social organization, and shared notions of authority and value" (Hendrickson 1996: 2). For Hildi Hendrickson fashion is a field for representation with semiotic value and social import. The value in question could be spiritual, economic, and/or political. When political, fashion can define a person or group in differentiation from another either as an expression of who they are, or still who they do not want to be, that is, fashion could participate in identity politics and the politics of resistance and/or representation.

For members of the Siphithemba Choir, their choice of fashion has multiple significances. Wicky Shabane, a female member of the choir, explained their choice of the *rainbow nation* colors as following what is in vogue, namely symbolic identification with the new South Africa. Her explanation is consistent with Elirea Bornman's finding in a study that was published in 2006 on nation-building in post-apartheid South Africa, which showed that support for rainbow nation symbolisms went hand in hand with national pride especially among Black South African groups (Bornman 2006: 383–399).

For Xolani Zulu who founded the African Vision fashion shop, their choices are conscious ways of projecting African identity, a process that is particularly important to them given South Africa's colonial and apartheid history in which dressing in Western styles was one of the ways in which Africans were subjugated. Under that history, those who wanted to be exempted from the culturally and socially alienating *bantu* laws were required to produce proof of literacy, pledge oath of allegiance, and lead lifestyle that reflected European civilization including conversion to the Christian faith and dressing in European fashion (see Davenport 2000 [1987]: 115). Thus the choir's fashion choice is both an expression of national pride and projection of Africanness. The choir uses the uniforms to project their African identity while reiterating Pan-African vision and ideological commitment to the African course. On another level, it is also a statement of resistance to some of the ways in which HIV/AIDS has been politicized both at the national and global scenes, a dynamic that has forced race and racial discourse upon the HIV/AIDS problem, whereby the African body became synonymous with the HIV/AIDS pandemic, an issue that I intend to address next in this chapter.

SIPHITHEMBA IN THE POLITICS OF REPRESENTATION

My first direct contact with the Siphithemba Choir was a meeting with Phumlani and Xolani, which took place in Xolani's African Vision Shop on West Street in the Durban Central Business District (CBD) in early May 2007. After several phone calls, Phumlani and I had arranged to meet at his office at the Center for AIDS Programme of Research in South Africa (CAPRISA) in Durban. On the scheduled date, Phumlani opted to meet me in front of the Durban Christian Centre, since, as he said, I might get confused trying to locate CAPRISA. Upon meeting, he told me that he had invited another member, one of his assistants, who oversees public-relations issues, to join us. The other person, I would later learn, was Xolani Zulu. We drove down to Xolani's African Vision Shop on West Street.

At the shop, Xolani and Phumlani asked that I explain to them what my mission was and what it was exactly that I wanted of the choir. After describing my research interest and specifying what I intended to document and how, Phumlani said, "You know, you're the first person to really show interest in our music." Xolani agreed that that was indeed the truth. I was surprised to hear them make such remark. I knew that the choir had toured abroad.

I wondered why people who had no interest in the choir's music would invite the choir overseas, so I asked them to explain what they meant.

Phumlani explained that a lot of their tours had been associated with the medical-science community. In many of these tours their primary audiences had been scientists who apparently believed that the members of the choir were living evidence of the success of their research. Xolani said that the scientists sometimes behaved as if they did not believe in God, and that they did not care about the choir members' sensibilities. He told the story of how one of the scientists had come backstage as the choir had been getting ready to perform at the Boston conference to alert them that they should not sing about God or Jesus on the stage. To avoid a conflict with the sponsors who had brought them to America, they began to make adjustments. Their song line-up for the event included some Zulu traditional songs, but it was packed with gospel songs. They quickly ran through their song titles and lyrics to ensure that none had explicit mention of God or Jesus, not in English or, even if in IsiZulu, at least not in a manner that is easily discernable by a non-Zulu speaker. One song however was bound to potentially create a problem for them. The song "Izizwe Maihlome" begins with the solo call "Nguyela uJesu" often led by Phumlani himself as soloist.

Phumlani explained that they had quickly altered the word *u-Jesu* in the song (see "Musical Adaptation" in chapter 6) to *uSomandla.* The irony, however, is that *uSomandla* in IsiZulu, meaning 'omnipotent,' is a title for God; since the scientific audience had not understood Zulu, they had not been offended, because they had not heard "God" or "Jesus," at least not in English.

The sense I got from this conversation was that the choir members had believed they were being exhibited as evidence of the success of medical research. As if telling me what they expected of me as a reciprocal gesture for studying with them, they indicated that they wished to travel anywhere and be able to perform their music to audiences that would be neutral to the political debates and disputes over treatments for AIDS. They wanted to sing for audiences who loved music and had ears to listen to their songs and hear their stories. In subsequent conversations with them, and through interviews with individual members, it became clear to me that, whereas they appreciate the opportunity to travel overseas to perform, they are nevertheless worried that their own story was being lost in the story of scientists' showcasing them as evidence of their research accomplishments.

The original motive behind the founding of the Siphithemba choir, the meaning of their songs, their spirituality, their social bonds, the microeconomic projects they ran to support themselves financially, their aspirations, their hopes, their determination to struggle with the virus together, all these things that had made them take the name *Siphithemba*, meaning 'We Give

Hope' or 'Give Us Hope', are being lost in the scientists' story, yet the scientists' story is not the story of the Siphithemba Choir.

The health sociologist Paula Treichler's theorizing about HIV/AIDS as "an epidemic of [meaning and] signification," (1999) speaks to how social and cultural processes and political dynamics account for the ways in which AIDS has been interpreted and how meanings have been constructed around the disease in local contexts and on the global scene. Her analysis also could help to explain the issue of the dynamics of the relationship between the choir and the scientific community, which in this chapter I argue as being symptomatic of the nature of the relationship between Africa and the West as it pertains to the politics of global health. I place the relationship dynamic and thus discuss it within the framework of the politics of representation, which scholars, using media reductionist reportages and health images of Africa, have observed as being intentional and purposeful: namely aimed at sustaining certain stereotypical images of Africa (Hall 2003), and to influence public policies and ultimately shape the modalities of Western response to disease epidemic in Africa (see McCombs and Shaw 1973; McCombs 1997; and Schraeder and Endless 1998: 29).

Stuart Hall (2003), drawing upon the semiotic and discursive ideas of Ferdinand de Saussure (1960) and the linguistic analysis of Michel Foucault (1980), argued about media as text and system of signs which shape ideas and concepts. Saussure posits language as a system of signs, namely the signifier and the signified, the relationships of which generate meanings via the merging of concepts with things or events, which they describe. Foucault on the other hand takes the linguistic model to another level, emphasizing discourse as a system of representation. Statements produce meaning through language. Foucault however introduced the idea of time as a modifying factor in discourse, in that the event may happen over a spaced timeframe over which certain discourse, like signs that signify, can evoke powerful meaning. Saussure's and Foucault's theories have informed literary and media critiques who watch the nature of representations of Africa in the West and who argue against the sustained reductionist images of the continent to their Western audiences. Stuart Hall notes, when it comes to images of Africa and the non-Western world, the meanings generated by the systems of signification created by the media are not dynamic; rather they tend to be fixed. Such manners of representation Schraeder and Endless argued in their 1998 essay, drawing upon the "agenda setting and framing" discourses of McCombs and Shaw (see McCombs and Shaw 1973; and McCombs 1997) sustains the National Geographic image of Africa, and which in turn shape public policies and Western response to disease epidemic in Africa (Schraeder and Endless 1998: 29).

With regard to the AIDS epidemic, Paula Treichler described the media representations as "Eurocentric, biased, doomsday Western AIDS coverage"

(1999: 209); wherein Africans at large are cast in the light as passive recipients of external aid (see Mwiinga 1993; Kalyango and Onyebadi 2012); too ignorant, too poor and so unsophisticated to understand how to deal with the exigencies of HIV/AIDS. In the light of these forms of media reportage, Treichler argues policy solutions are offered that overlook the sociocultural realities on the ground; and Western pharmaceutical companies find critical mass of promising population for vaccine experimentations and testing.

Whereas the scientist do not necessarily control the media, they always hold the gaze of the cameras of media corporations, world leaders, and big money donors, all of whom are vital to the public representations of the works of the community, and/or who bring the money to sustain their research. In a conversation with Zinhle Thabethe, the female member of the choir who gave the keynote speech at the Boston conference, she noted,

> being there on the stage with [former] President Bill Clinton, with all the media and the eyes of the world on us was big for me. So I thought if I am going to do this [the keynote speech], I better do it well because, maybe I will never have the opportunity again to tell them about us.

In other words, for Zinhle, the platform of the stage was the most opportune time to introduce her own story and the story of her choir members as distinctive and apart from the story the scientists wanted the world to hear. I therefore suggest in this chapter that Siphithemba's story is a narrative of self-representation, aimed at subverting the appropriation of their story by the scientific community who showcase them as evidence of their scientific accomplishment. Furthermore, a brief examination of the contextual encounters of the choir members with American audiences during their tours also suggests that the choir has a consciousness of themselves as engaging in the campaign of counter-narrative in the HIV/AIDS discourse that paints the disease in a one-sided light as solely an African problem.

COMPETING NARRATIVES AND CONTESTED OWNERSHIP OF THE SUCCESS STORIES

In chapter 2 I discussed how by 1998, the success of the HIV/AIDS project at McCord Hospital was drawing international attention, informing thus the decision to erect a special AIDS clinic there, and how the Siphithemba Choir which had already been formed was readily deployed to help raise funds for the clinic by performing at major events at the hospital and around Durban. Since Harvard Medical School was involved in erecting of the clinic, especially because the hospital served as a testing site for a CD4/Viral Load research project, sponsored by the Center for AIDS Research at the Massachusetts General Hospital and Harvard Medical School, and given that many of the Sinikithemba Support Group members were participants in the project under the leadership of Professor Bruce Walker, the choir directly became involved with the scientific community. Again, it was Professor Walker who oversaw the choir's second tour in 2003 for the purposes of participating in the Boston Conference on Retroviruses and Opportunistic Infections, followed by several other oversea tours in the United States and Britain.

Whereas these oversea tours enabled the choir to forge closer ties with the scientific community, boosted their economic well-being, as well as raised their profile back home in South Africa, the new relationship with the scientific community also revealed some degree of contention about who gets the credit for the achievements of the choir and the members physical healthiness manifest in the exuberant music and dance performances. This contention is evidenced in the demand during the Boston conference that the choir must not perform any song about God on the stage. The demand was made irrespective of the fact that the choir is part of a mission hospital, was founded first and foremost as a support group with prayer and spiritual counseling at the center of their activities, and that hymns and gospel songs predominate in their repertoires. According to the choir director Phumlani Kunene, this demand by the scientists was condescending, patronizing, and amounted to utter disregard of the fact that their music is a means of telling their own story and not the story of the scientists.

The truth is that medical research on AIDS did not give birth to the Siphithemba Choir; rather, the members' desire to support one another in their struggles with the virus, their determination to beat the odds of being HIV-positive, and their effort to bring the message of hope and educate their community in the same vein account for the formation of the ensemble. Hence, although the members have benefited in their relationship with the medical researchers, they still desire to control the message so that their story becomes paramount in the circumstances of that relationship.

It is therefore arguable that the story of the relationship of the Siphithemba Choir with the scientists is symptomatic—when viewed at least from the perspective of choir members—of the West's patronizing relationship with Africa. There is a seeming assumption—perhaps unconscious—by Westerners who embark on humanitarian and research efforts in Africa that Africans are, as previously stated, helpless and incapable of finding solutions to their problems. Hence Africa becomes according to Treichler the critical space for vaccine experimentations and drug testing. When these experiments fail, Africans, who comprise the majority of the subjects, suffer. An example is the reported case of a microbicide gel manufactured by an American pharmaceutical company, a potential treatment that failed in KwaZulu-Natal in 2007 and infected many young Zulu women with HIV (Skoler-Karpoff 2008: 1977–1987, see also Howden 2009). When success has been recorded, however, the rules of patents and costs have made it extremely difficult for Africans to gain access to the drugs. At other times, estern scientists instigate doubts about Africans' ability to handle complicated drug regimens such as the antiretroviral regimen because of ignorance about the use of drugs. Choir member Zinhle Thabethe who gave the keynote during the tenth annual Conference on Retroviruses and Opportunistic Infections in Boston rebutted this argument, offering herself as a living example of the success of antiretrovirals in an African environment, thanks to her diligence and ability to manage the complexity of the regimen (Hainsworth 2006).

Given Zinhle's ability to use the platform of the concert stage to respond to Western scientists' patronizing attitudes, it seems the choir can still meet its objective of raising its voice and telling their own story without necessarily letting them be subsumed in that of the scientific community who want to showcase the choir as evidence of the success of their research endeavors. The problem though is that they lack the platform to do so on a regular basis and with the possibility of wide dissemination of their story such as through media channels. As a choral ensemble, they are also known for their performance of music about HIV/AIDS; hence they are sometimes called an AIDS choir. As a result, only those who have personal interest and/or are stakeholders in the AIDS issue are drawn to their story. It is difficult for them to break out of this stereotype. They lack the resources to mobilize for overseas concert tours without sponsorships from medical researchers and AIDS philanthropists, who draw a specific type of audience because of the work they do.

In contrast however, given Zinhle's ability to use the platform of the concert stage to respond to Western scientists' patronizing attitudes, it seems the choir can still meet its objective of raising its voices in respect of their experience of HIV/AIDS without necessarily separating from the medical science community. The choir had opportunities to tour schools and churches each time it visited the United States, where its members educate non-science audiences by narrating their personal experiences.

Regarding the scientist's demand that the choir refrain from singing about God and Jesus on stage, the choir subverted that restriction through the use of language. Textual redaction and manipulation of language are ways in which Black South Africans resisted apartheid (Kivnick 1990: 326; Detterbeck 2002: 150). Siphithemba, for its part, has used language ingeniously, as shown in chapter 6. It creatively manages circumstances similar to the one at the Boston conference.

In the end, it might well be the case that Siphithemba is concerned about being "re-presented" in an objectifying manner as the results of scientific research, rather than being granted the benefit to be self-represented as human subjects with agency. Its members can represent themselves and narrate their stories even within the environment where they perceive themselves as being dehumanized. The probable question, then, is what effect does this paradoxical modes of representation have on their foreign audiences?

"WE ARE POSITIVE TOO": HIV/AIDS AS EQUALLY WESTERN ISSUE

The members of the Siphithemba Choir believe that when they are on tour in North America, part of their mission is to raise awareness about the AIDS crisis in (South) Africa, and to raise funds to support the course of treatment and prevention. In many of their tours, they visited churches and local schools, where they addressed issues related to their individual experiences and those of their communities back home through performance. In conversation with Dr. Bruce Walker, I learned that the choir's school visits had prompted students in some schools in the Boston area to start their own projects for propagating an AIDS- awareness campaign. Dr. Walker stated that the first tour sponsored by the Church World Services was organized to "help them increase their exposure so people can see the faces of the people we've been turning our backs on" (*Boston Globe* 2003). For him, it is important to put a human face on a disease that has often been reduced to statistics.

It appears that the sensibilities of the choir in terms of their spirituality, hope, and resilience are not lost on their American audiences. For instance, the Church World Service newsletter of spring 2003, a special edition with the theme "War and Peace," reported that the choir's "tour sought to raise resources for and awareness about the AIDS crisis in Africa, and to vividly convey the beauty, courage, and creativity of the people of Africa" (2003:12). Other reports from the newsletter described how the choir's performances, which began at the Riverside Church in New York City on World AIDS Day and concluded in Washington D.C., "evoked the enthusiastic responses in each of their eleven concert venues," commonly accompanied with standing ovations and tears.

The emotionality of the responses in the churches could have been for different reasons. It is often easy for AIDS to be discussed in North America as an African or developing-world problem. Some people who are infected or affected by HIV and AIDS in America tend to live in denial of their individual experience of AIDS. While most of the reporting and commentaries on the choir's tours reiterate the increased awareness that the group brought about the AIDS crisis in Africa, the choir members made observations about Americans who are HIV-positive but have difficulty disclosing their status. In the Church World Service newsletter of spring 2003, an unnamed choir member remarked:

> We notice that Americans who are HIV+ were very shy about telling others they had AIDS. We would be just about to leave and then someone would come forward and quickly tell us that they were HIV+. We think that perhaps we were role models for Americans living with AIDS and that maybe we helped some of them to think about being more open about their status. We hope we have given them confidence. (2003: 13)

It appears from the nature of these interactions, that some Americans who have HIV or AIDS are still less likely to reveal that fact than many people in South Africa. A few years ago, it was reported on National Public Radio that about half the Americans who ought to submit to HIV testing refuse to do so, suggesting that the actual number of Americans living with HIV and AIDS may never be known. The November 2014 supplemental report issued by the Center for Disease Control stated: "Over the past decade, the number of people living with HIV has increased, while the annual number of new HIV infections has remained relatively stable. Still, the pace of new infections continues at far too high a level."[9] According to the report, of the number of people living with HIV infection, one in seven are unaware of their status. This lack of awareness is compounded by the refusal of individuals to submit to testing, thanks to the stigmatization of HIV/AIDS, which is still high and strong in the United States. The reality of the stigma is captured in the testimony of an anonymous young female:

> By now you'd think people would know a lot about HIV, but they don't. Even when I do feel close enough to someone . . . , I wonder. The truth is that people really do look at you differently when they know you are HIV positive. . . . It is hard. But I know people's ignorance is not going to go away. I still think people are going to hate me or not want to be my friend when they learn I have HIV. (DeNoon 2009)

To some people who bear the burden of the stigma of AIDS in the United States therefore, the Siphithemba Choir offers hope and courage through its performances. Such individuals recognize that they share common experiences with members of the choir, and they are moved to extend a hand of solidarity with the group. By so doing, they gain spiritual and emotional strength to confront their fears and accept their situation. Thus, Siphithemba's music is not only well received for moving their American audiences to appreciate their experience of HIV/AIDS and to extend hands of charity toward

Africans with AIDS, they are equally successful in awakening a new level of consciousness about AIDS within American society.

SUMMARY AND CONCLUSION

The issue of the politics of HIV/AIDS is more than just a question of "structural violence" (Farmer 2005: 20–40) that is steeped in social and economic inequities that exists in socieities. This work with the Siphithemba Choir and a close reading of their songs and activities reveal multifaced aspects of the politics of global health and the HIV/AIDS in particular. The politics is about differentials in culture, faith, and knowledge, as it is about economic and social capital. These issues though often imagined to operate outside of the domains of public health, nevertheless are intertiwined, and they filter into and become defining factors in how people interact in the domain of health. In the case of the Siphithemba Choir it all played out on both local and international scenes, leaving one to wonder (at least at the face value) why issues of racial and ethic identity would preoccupy a group of individuals who are battling with a more serious health issue. The truth is, their activities and approach to the issues are partly in response to the ways in which they, Africans, and Africa has been portayed in the grand discourses on the global AIDS epidemic. Hence theirs is a conscious type of counter-narrative to the more common ways in which Africa and Africans have been represented in the discourse as helpless and passive reciepients of aid in the context of disease epidemic. It is a narrative of health that runs contrary to the image of Africa being projected to the world; they are also an example of a proactive African response to local issues that rarely form part of mainstream media reportage on Africa.

It is possible that the choir's use of music and dance and the concert stage has the potential to to reinforce the exotic stereotypical images of Africa that are rooted in the nineteenth-century ethnological show business (see Lindfors 1999: vii). I suggest however, that even if any such exotic curiosity may have been elicited by their performances to foreign audience, it has equally been successful in letting them add their voices to the conversations on AIDS treatment as well as helped to reveal the reality of HIV/AIDS in the American and western society that is often not acknowledged in a rather often one-sided view narrative of the global HIV/AIDS problem (see Okigbo and Ezumah 2015:15).

NOTES

1. See also the CDC fast facts "HIV in the United States: *At A Glance.*" *Center for Disease Control.* http://www.cdc.gov/hiv/statistics/basics/ataglance.html cited November 28, 2014.

2. For details on how the nature of HIV genomes and its regional distribution may have impacted the experience of the choir members and why it found expression in their music, see Okigbo, Austin C. 2011: 241–51.

3. For more on this see Fassin 2007: 161–168.

4. President Thabo Mbeki for instance was known to sometimes instigate the racial reading of the South African experience of HIV/AIDS by constantly referencing the link between apartheid and the pandemic. In doing so he created an atmosphere of antagonism between his administration and the White liberal media and scientists whose Black colleagues often defended Mbeki's position and "sometimes expressed irritation at the attacks against him (Fassin 2007: 10–11).

5. Bantu Education was crafted by the apartheid state for Black South Africans as a way to keep them from upward economic and social mobility. According to Wilfrid Cardinal Napier, the Cardinal Archbishop of Durban, the very first Good Friday Ecumenical liturgy was organized behind the prison where the priests were detained and was led by late Archbishop Denis Hurley of Durban.

6. Other Black composers' choral works that manifest a similar nationalist tone use terms such as *abanssundu* and *abamnyama,* both of which mean 'black'; sometimes these other words are used interchangeably with *Africa.*

7. *Umfundisi* in Zulu means 'priest' (or 'father,' as in the case of a Catholic priest) or 'teacher,' depending on the tonal accent. Siphithemba members know that I am a Roman Catholic priest, so they sometimes call me by my first name, and other times they just call me *umfundisi.*

8. Wax prints are colorful clothing fabrics widely worn by women in West Africa (also found in Central and East Africa). Originally produced in Holland, and now in Nigeria and Ghana, the fabrics have paintings of human figures and assorted images with inscriptions that convey messages about ethnic, and sometimes gender identity.

9. *HIV Surveillance Supplemental Report* 2014; 19 (No. 3). http://www.cdc.gov/hiv/library/reports/surveillance/ (accessed on March 10, 2015).

Chapter 9

Conclusion

Reflections on Siphithemba Choir and the Politics of AIDS and Health

Ethnography on music and HIV/AIDS (and health in general) has tended to focus largely on the use of music in creating awareness and as grassroots mobilization for disease prevention. The persistence of this type of writing once again became manifest during the 2014 ebola outbreak in three West African countries as exemplified in Linda Poon's article on the musical activities in Liberia and Sierra Leone aimed at eliciting public conversations on the new "state of emergency" (Poon 2014). When ethnographic work has addressed issues of politics on the other hand it has mostly been about activism, and in the case of HIV/AIDS in (South) Africa, it's largely about countering cultural practices and/or public policies that exacerbate the problem or mitigate the containment of disease.

At the beginning of my study in South Africa, there was one major thing I sought to learn about in addition to grassroots musical awareness campaigns and activism that were already ubiquitous in public media. I wanted to know if and how much the music of the antiapartheid struggles may have been transformed, reinterpreted, and redeployed in the ongoing fight against HIV/AIDS. Although this type of musical activity was evident, my perspective broadened if not changed whence I began working with the Siphithemba Choir. I realized that as a group of individuals who are HIV-positive, their knowledge of the local and global cultural and political dynamics that impinge upon people's experiences of the virus is much more sophisticated than people in their positions are often given credit for in Africa. Through their style of organizing, musical processes and stylistics, they engage as well as address the cultural and political manifestations of HIV/AIDS at multiple levels—individual and group, local, and transnational.

My use of the method of micro-analyses in this study, an approach that seeks to understand the big picture of social issues through careful examination of small or specific case study of social processes and/or communicative (and performance) behavior (Le Baron 2006), allowed me to place the choir and the cultural and political issues their music portends to engage in the broader context of South Africa's public health and political history, and the global, albeit transnational culture and politics of HIV/AIDS. In the end, what I learned is that HIV/AIDS is the most politicized public-health issue of our time, both nationally and internationally with the capacity to generate varied levels of sociocultural productions and policy debates. Also, although local communities and national policymakers tend to forge solutions to the HIV/AIDS problem in accordance with their unique situations, yet, the local sometimes is reflective of the global, just as much as the global has a place in the local.

In this study therefore, I have underscored the importance of an ethnographic approach and framework that takes into account the specificities of local contexts, and the worldviews and sensibilities of my research collaborators. I also tried to underscore how their worldviews and their individual and collective experiences defined the musical choices of the choir and how they use their music to both articulate those experiences and to engage the local and global discourses on HIV/AIDS. My ethnographic study of the Siphithemba Choir is a case study of a local response to HIV/AIDS, informed by unique individual and group experiences, and the historical circumstances of local and national politics. In examining the choir's use of choral music as an expressive form of engaging HIV/AIDS, I have situated the choir within the larger historical context of Zulu and South African musical performance as a site of expression of struggle, expressions of social, economic, and political aspirations, contestations of power, and responses to societal problems including issues of public health.

In South Africa, apartheid and its economic, social, and political practices have been largely identified as the major contributing factor to the rapidity of the spread of HIV/AIDS within the African population (de Gruchy and de Gruchy 2005; Fassin 2007; Gilbert and Walker 2002; Hunt 1996; Jochelson and Leger 1991). Hence, when former president Nelson Mandela declared HIV/AIDS "the next struggle," triggering a new connection of the current fight with that of the antiapartheid struggle, people naturally responded to the disease with the same spirit that characterized their struggle against apartheid. Christian churches in particular responded by resorting to the same tools that had aided them in the fight against apartheid: the intellectual groundwork in the form of Black Theology and the Black Consciousness Movement, grassroots movements in the form of protest liturgy, and community-based income-generating projects for poverty alleviation. On a broader societal level, the indigenous Nguni *Ubuntu* philosophy that emphasized community and human interconnection and mutual interdependency has been invoked as a means to mobilize the nation against the onslaught of the disease and the social fallouts such as stigma. The philosophy itself got a unique interpretation and functional applicability with the Siphithemba Choir and as a support group who recognized the importance of working together and by engaging in industry as a means to earn a living and be responsible citizens and meaningful contributors to the good of the larger society. The application of the philosophy also is apparent in their communal approach to song composition and musical performances.

On another level, just as music comprised an integral part of the antiapartheid struggle, it has become a major tool in the fight against HIV/AIDS. I have seen in the course of my research how, many of the songs have since been transformed, adapted, and reinterpreted to address the experience of the HIV/AIDS pandemic. In a similar vein, the Siphithemba Choir, in addition to composing its own songs, continues to adapt and reinterpret pre-existing traditional and gospel songs to address their individual, group, and community experiences of HIV/AIDS.

The connections thus made raise questions about the relationship of people and the larger perspectives of faith, health, the arts, and science within the levels of analysis laid out in this work. The Siphithemba Choir, by virtue of being founded in a mission hospital, and for the preponderance of church hymns and gospel music in their repertoire may be considered a faith-based group: it embodies and exemplifies the effects of faith-based initiatives in confronting issues that affect local communities. It comprises a convergence of church efforts at empowering people at the grassroots levels through prayer and industry. Its success in the fight against HIV/AIDS, engaged within the space of a mission hospital, reiterates the notion about faith-based health assets, premised on the notion that "a church that takes preferential option for the health of the [person] is a church faithful to the healing and wholeness implied by the Latin word *salus,* from which we derive 'salvation'" (Cochraine 2006: 18).

The laudable works of the faith-based health initiatives notwithstanding, issues of boundaries and barriers (Cochraine 2006) call for interrogation. My encounter with Zanele at a support-group meeting (discussed in chapter 1) comes to mind here. How does one reconcile an infected person's expression of Christian faith with his or her advocacy of preventive measures (e.g., the use of condoms) that are proscribed by sectarian doctrines, which see such measures as contrary to the dictates of the Christian faith, or even as conveniences that encourage promiscuity? When Roger Cardinal Mahony, former archbishop of Los Angeles declared on CNN that the high rate of HIV/AIDS in sub-Saharan Africa is being fueled by sexual promiscuity, I wondered whether his utterance showed an ecclesiastical disconnect with the reality of HIV/AIDS within its own communal body. Such utterances, I argued in chapter 5, only fuel the stigmatizing of people living with AIDS, making them double victims of the virus. Progressive theologians and churchmen, such as Bishop Kevin Dowling of Rustenburg,[1] South Africa, who called on the Roman Catholic Church to permit the use of condoms so as to stop "transmitting death" (TRC Report, January 2002) may have stirred the ire of the Vatican, yet the controversy that followed his statement indicates an ecclesiastical ambivalence in a social gospel that emphasizes "embracing those desperately in need of God's love in action" (Meadows 2003: 151). I say this of course without prejudice to Pope Benedict XVI's rather tepid suggestion in 2010 that condom use by male prostitutes could comprise an important first step to individual responsibility in preventing the spread of HIV.[2] Like Zanele, the members of the Siphithemba Choir are quite aware of the ambivalence inherent in Christian social teachings on HIV/AIDS. As people living with HIV and AIDS, waiting for a change in the doctrine of the church so as to be accepted and to work aggressively toward disease prevention is not an option. The choir may not have the privilege of the pulpit, but as a touring music group, it came to possess the power of the concert stage, from which to proclaim its members' own version of the gospel of social justice and the right to life.

A question that might follow is: which bodies have priority here? The discussions in this work show that the Siphithemba Choir, along with certain voices in the public-policy debates (including former president Thabo Mbeki), chose to answer the question in racial terms. It is Africans, isolated by the Western scientific community as the originators of the virus, and found by Western scientists to be a promising population for vaccine experimentations and testing (Treichler 2004: 209). Yet it is Africans who were long denied access to the appropriate antiretroviral regimen. In South Africa from the late apartheid era to date, Black Africans have been neglected in public health-care (Nattrass in 2007; Seftel 1988; Viljoen 1989); they were deported to neighboring countries when the apartheid state decided to implement a policy on HIV/AIDS. Black Africans were still denied (until recently) antiretroviral drugs and the mother-to-child prevention drug—ironically, by a Black-led administration in a post-apartheid democratic state. One is bound to be curious how HIV/AIDS has come to embody the nature of the asymmetry between the North and the South, especially between Africa and the West, the haves and the have-nots, White and Black. While the economic and social disparities between the two worlds—the West and Africa—still abound, one wonders whether the right to a just distribution of healthcare would become the decisive leveling factor in global affairs. How that would play out may not be certain, but we get a clue from the legal battle that was fought between the South African government and the major multinational pharmaceutical giants. By seeking to bypass international patent laws to produce generic forms of the antiretrovirals in 2005, South Africa under Thabo Mbeki forced the Western pharmaceutical companies to lower the cost of the drugs drastically, and this move is largely responsible for increased dissemination of the drugs across Africa and other third-world countries.

Mbeki's legal maneuver is not inconsistent with his idea that gave birth to the New Partnership for Africa's Development, which is couched in the ideology of the African Renaissance. The idea is about Africa's self-determination without being tied to the terms of foreign aid. It is consistent with the objectives of the Siphithemba Choir when it sings in "Siyaphela Isizwe seNkosi" that Africa must rise to fight the pandemic. It is the same idea that was behind their objective when Mrs. Mhlongo said, "What we are trying to inculcate to people is that they have to work and not beg. Because of their [HIV/AIDS] status, they shouldn't go around begging."

The choir's sense of self-determination has therefore played out on different levels: on the economic level by virtue of engaging in skills acquisition and working to earn a living, and by utilizing concert tours to boost incomes above the South African poverty index. It has played out internationally by turning concert stages into platforms for speaking out against the denial of access to appropriate drugs just because the people who need those drugs are Black Africans. Also, as discussed earlier in the preceding chapter, despite its openness to working with the scientific community, the Siphithemba Choir maintains that as a group of individuals who live the experience of being HIV-positive, their collective story is distinct from that of the scientists. The choir members want to tell their own stories in the way that they see fit—primarily through their music.

It is important therefore for ethnographic purposes, that ethnography of AIDS music in Africa recognize that the global has a place in the local. In South Africa, the national scene comprises a local space where different elements of the global politics of AIDS are played out. Local and global contexts have thus affected Siphithemba's organization and shaped how its perspective on HIV/AIDS is expressed in music. As I have argued, their quest for self-representation as opposed to being presented to the donor communities as evidence of the success of Western scientific research informs Siphithemba's performance of its members' experience of the virus as a counter-narrative, being as such a form of resistance. It is an original and local way of dealing with the disease.

On a final note, I am well aware of how and why my approach to the study of music and AIDS in South Africa, using the case study of the Siphithemba Choir, may be construed as falling into the trap of what the cultural theorist Sarah Nuttal of the University of Witwatersrand has described as post-apartheid writing with "neo-Marxist inflection" (2009). Nuttal has argued that by employing categories of race, class, domination and resistance in much the same way as critics had done in the decade or so before, "the dominant critical impulse tends to assert continuity with the past, producing a critique based on reiteration and return, and an argument in the name of that which has not changed in the country" (2009: 17). Inasmuch as I take cognizance of Nuttal's theorizing, I believe that an attempt to avoid what she argued as theoretical pitfall would amount to sidestepping the historical and political realities that contributed to the spread of the virus in the first place, and which continues to shape the AIDS discourse in South Africa. I highlighted a number of South African scholars especially scholars of social medicine who point to the historical roots of current public health challenges in South Africa. Coovadia H. and Jewkes R. (2009) for example pointed to the lingering effects of apartheid and how the current public health challenges are rooted in the historical legacies of apartheid. Another South African scholar of social medicine and public health Abdool Karim (2009) echoing the voices of earlier scholars (Brummer 2002; Jochelson 1991) points at the migrant labor system under apartheid, with its associated overcrowded male hostels and squatter settlements and deliberately underdeveloped health services for Blacks, as "providing a favourable environment for efficient transmission of HIV." My research reveals that these historical realities do filter into public and private conversations on the state of public health in South Africa in general and HIV/AIDS in particular. It means then that people's experience of HIV/AIDS is linked to their historical sociocultural and political experiences, thereby constituting the lens through which HIV/AIDS is viewed and interpreted.

When it comes to the ethnography of AIDS music therefore, and in the light of the works of scholars of social medicine and epidemiology that I have outlined above, I suggest that we pay attention to the kind of identity consciousness (be it racial, ethnic, or gender, etc.) that pervades the music of those who live the experience of being HIV/AIDS positive. It is important that we understand the historical and social realities that inform that consciousness, and how that consciousness conversely informs people's ways of responding to health situations.

In South Africa, the nature of the HIV/AIDS virus, the facts of the historical past, and the global politics of AIDS all impinge upon the various discourses interrogating AIDS in the context of public health. The Siphithemba Choir that is the subject of this study is a group of individuals who live the experience of being HIV-positive. As Black South Africans whose experiences have been shaped by the history of apartheid, the choir through their music therefore provide insights useful to understanding the social and cultural realities of AIDS in South Africa; they could be equally useful to understanding those realities the length and breadth of the continent and beyond.

In conclusion, I hope that I have added a new layer to the ethnography of AIDS music in (South) Africa. Studies on music and AIDS have focused largely on education through the use of arts and music as entertainment otherwise known as edutainment (Bourgault 2003; Rhafaldt 2007); as the communication of messages for disease prevention and care (Barz 2006; Bourgault 2003; Lwanda 2003; Rahfaldt 2007; Vaughan et al. 2000; etc.), and as healing (Barz 2006; Barz and Cohen 2008). There is a general recognition of the use of music as a form of activism, especially with regard to influencing public policy, as exemplified in the 46664 concerts. In all of these, little attention is paid to the issue of historicity and continuity in the use of musical performance, both as political discourse and in the challenge of public health. In addition to articulating the educational and communicative use of music, this book adds a layer of history to the study by inscribing the Siphithemba Choir in the Black choral-music tradition, which has been deployed on different fronts of the members' struggle experience. Unlike the other studies cited, this work brings choral music into an arena that has been devoted largely to popular music and popular culture.

By setting my study against the historical background of the human struggles in South Africa, and by linking the organization and performance of choral music in the current struggle with HIV/AIDS to creative antecedents in the historical challenges of human rights and public health, I have tried to negotiate the web of issues that have shaped Siphithemba's music and vision. Culture and the politics of culture, identity and race relations, faith, health, economic development, human rights, and public policy are often compartmentalized as separate domains of academic inquiry, yet the issues are interconnected. And there is perhaps no single issue that has caused these to collide or converge as much as the current global AIDS pandemic. Similarly, South Africa and its AIDS experience comprise a single territory, where this complex web of human activities is playing out.

Siphithemba, as I have tried to show, embodies this reality, and the choir members have embraced it as it is—in their vision, organization, and musical performance. If it has helped them deal with their experience of HIV and AIDS (and I believe it has), then studying them and discussing their music within the web of relevant issues is a worthy enterprise. It is further proof of the realization by scholars (Campbell 1997, 2000, 2003; Campbell and Williams 1999, Farmer 1997, 1999, 2003; Gottlieb 1990; Kauffman 2004; Nattrass 2007; and Treichler 2004) that HIV/AIDS must not be treated as an exclusively public-health problem. Whereas social, economic, political, environmental, and even religious factors affect people's experience of HIV/AIDS, so also do people respond to that experience from various angles of their modes of existence. The angles of their mode of being and responses to those experiences challenge us ethnographers to consider whether we want to treat the musical response to AIDS as a single string of action, or as part of a complex web of activities. For me, and in this work, I have chosen to treat it like the silver thread woven among, and through the fabrics of other threads of human activities.

NOTES

1. See also a statement by Carlo Maria Cardinal Martini, the former archbishop of Milan, printed in the Italian weekly *L'Espresso* and quoted in Boustany (2006).

2. See Donadio, Rachel and Goodstein, Laurie. November 20, 2010. "In Rare Cases, Pope Justifies Use of Condoms." In *New York Times* (http://www.nytimes.com/2010/11/21/world/europe/21pope.html?pagewanted=all&_r=0).

Appendix

Siphithemba Song, "Siyaphela Isizwe SeNkosi."

SIYAPHELA ISIZWE SENKOSI

Music by: Siphithemba Choir
Lyrics by: Phumulani & Sizwe

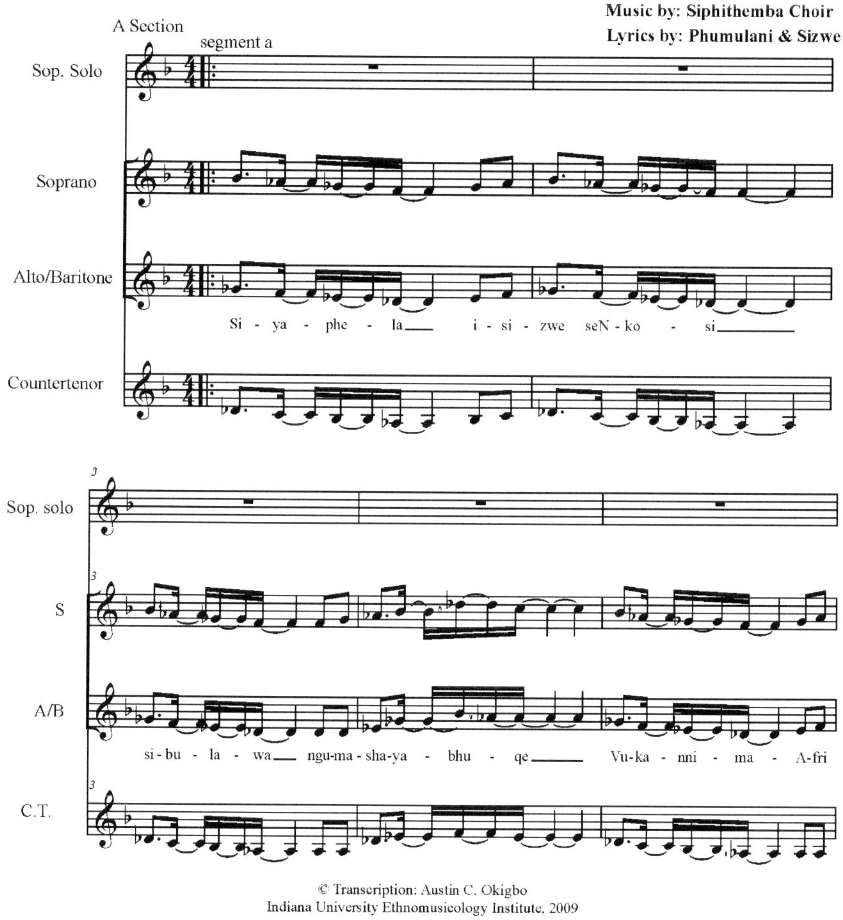

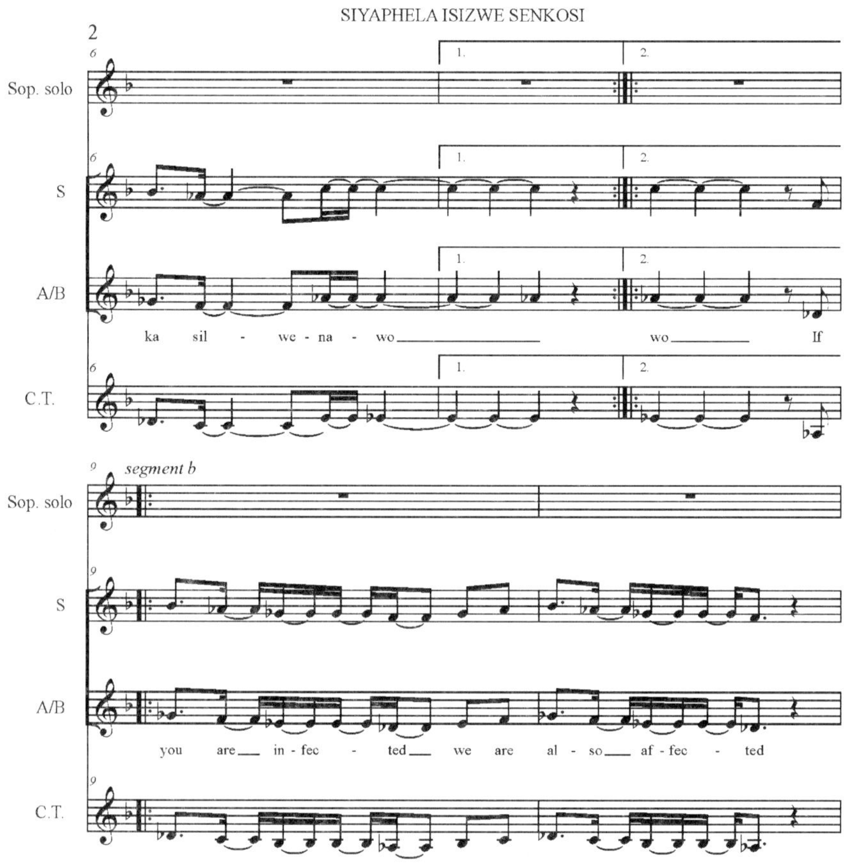
SIYAPHELA ISIZWE SENKOSI
2
Sop. solo
S
A/B
C.T.
1.
2.
ka sil - we - na - wo wo If
segment b
you are in - fec - ted we are al - so af - fec - ted

SIYAPHELA ISIZWE SENKOSI

3

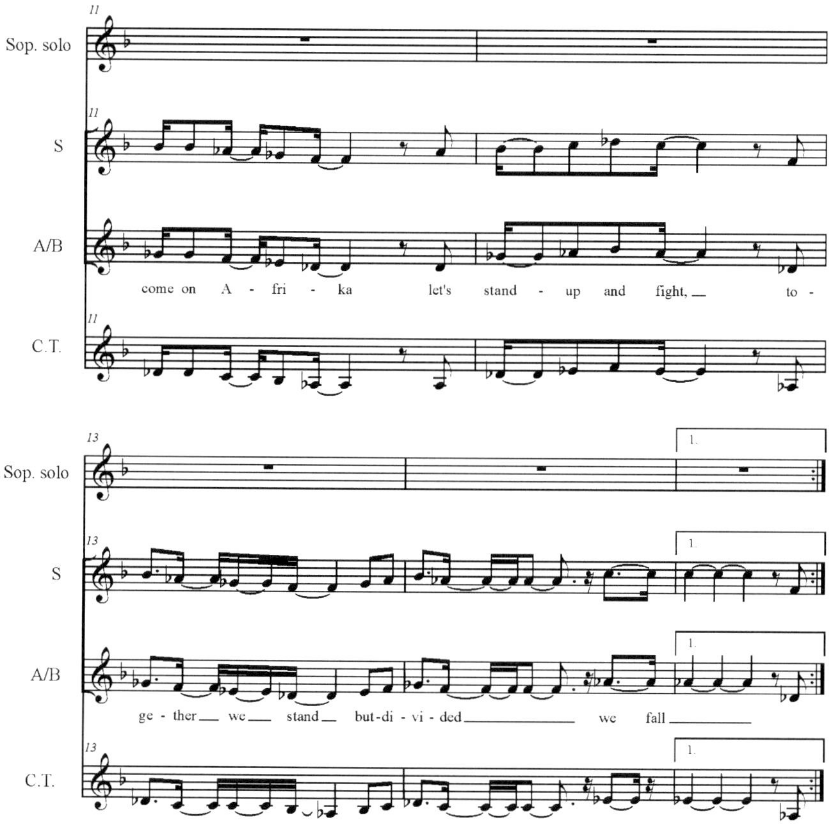
Sop. solo
S
A/B
C.T.
come on A - fri - ka let's stand - up and fight, to -
ge - ther we stand but-di - vi - ded we fall
1.

SIYAPHELA ISIZWE SENKOSI

4

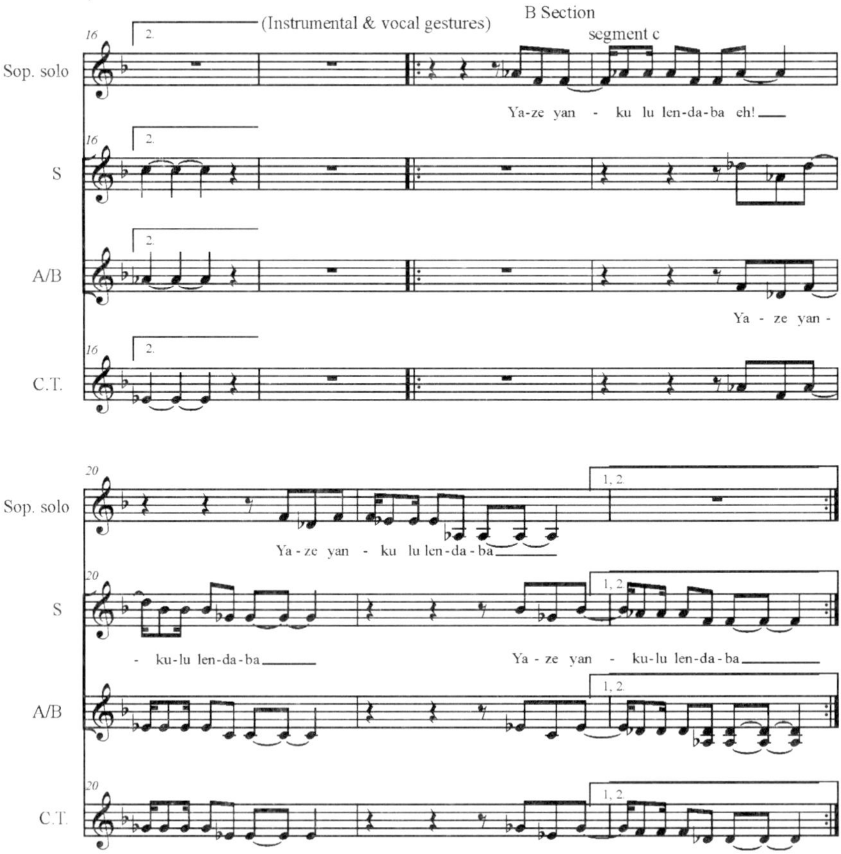

SIYAPHELA ISIZWE SENKOSI

5

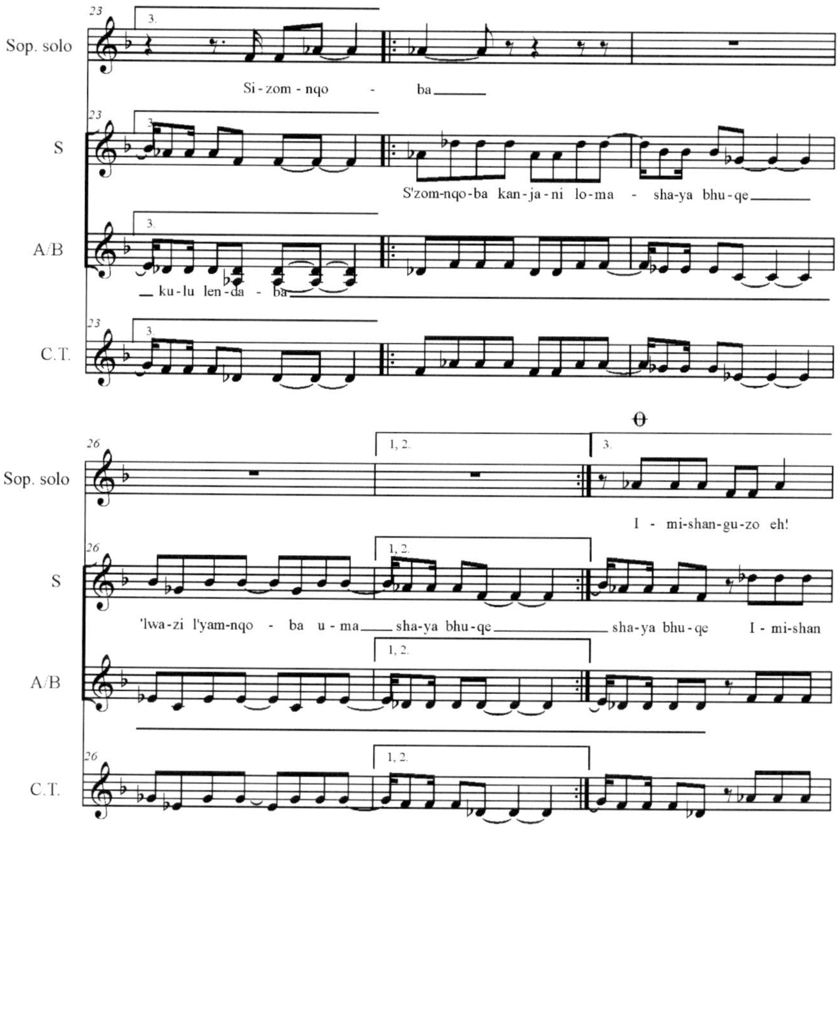
Sop. solo
S
A/B
C.T.
Si - zom - nqo - ba
S'zom-nqo-ba kan - ja - ni lo-ma - sha-ya bhu-qe
ku-lu len-da - ba
'lwa-zi l'yam-nqo - ba u - ma sha-ya bhu-qe sha-ya bhu-qe I - mi-shan
I - mi-shan-gu-zo eh!

SIYAPHELA ISIZWE SENKOSI

6

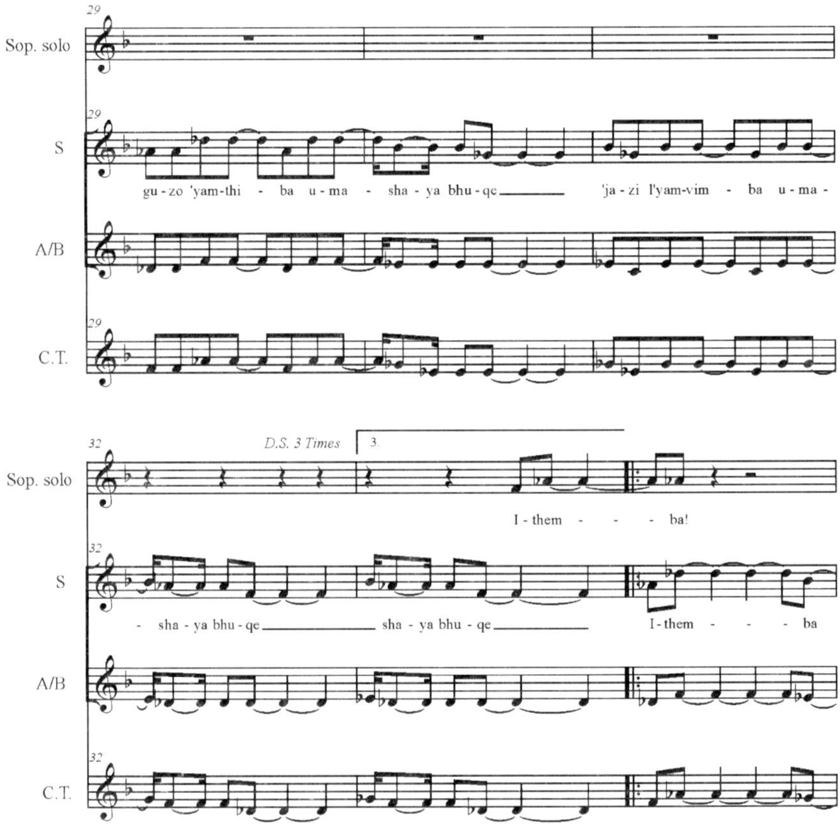

SIYAPHELA ISIZWE SENKOSI

7

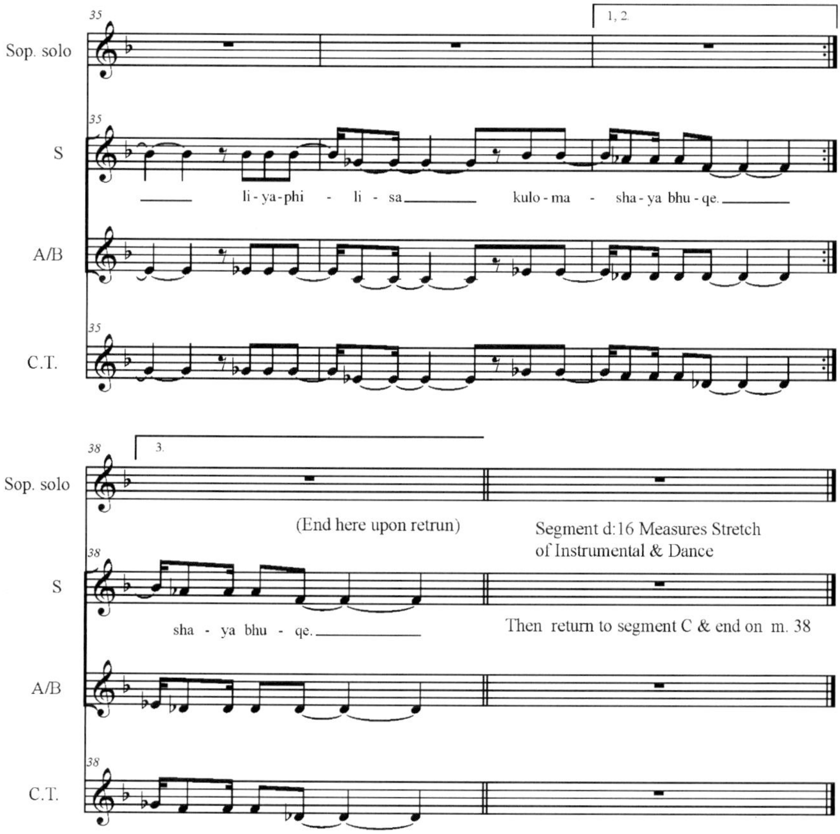
35
1, 2.
Sop. solo
S
li - ya - phi - li - sa kulo - ma - sha - ya bhu - qe.
A/B
C.T.
38
3.
Sop. solo
(End here upon retrun)
Segment d:16 Measures Stretch
of Instrumental & Dance
S
sha - ya bhu - qe.
Then return to segment C & end on m. 38
A/B
C.T.

Siphithemba Song, "Know Your Status."

YOU'VE GOT TO KNOW YOUR STATUS

Phumulani Kunene
[Siphithemba Choir]

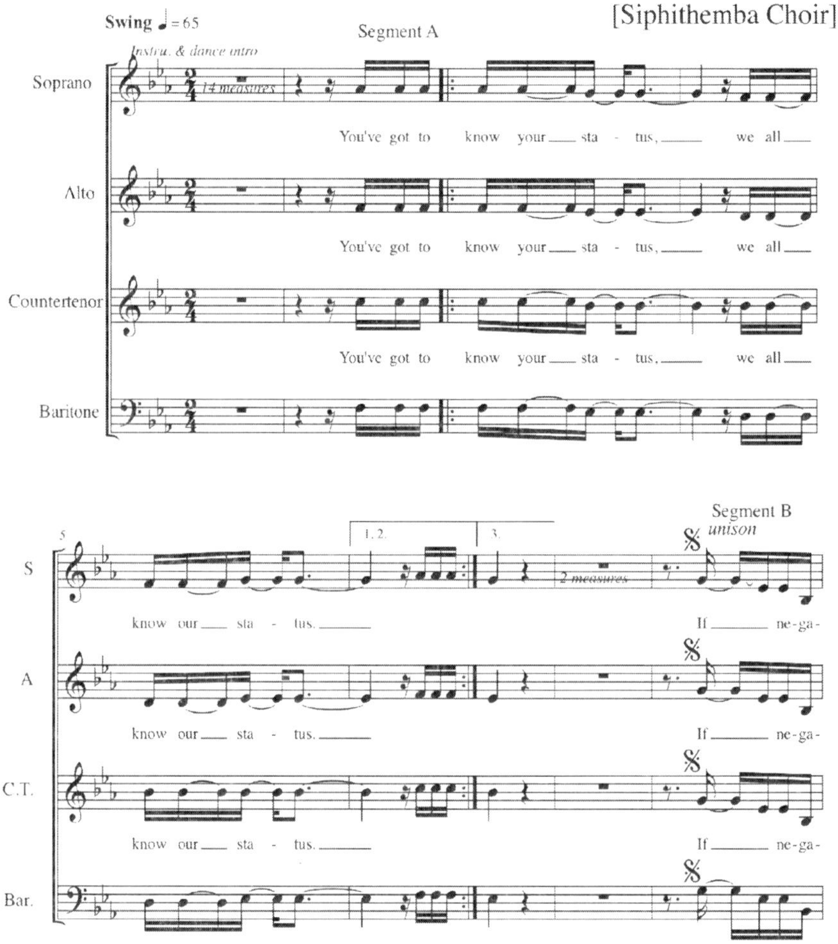

YOU'VE GOT TO KNOW YOUR STATUS 2

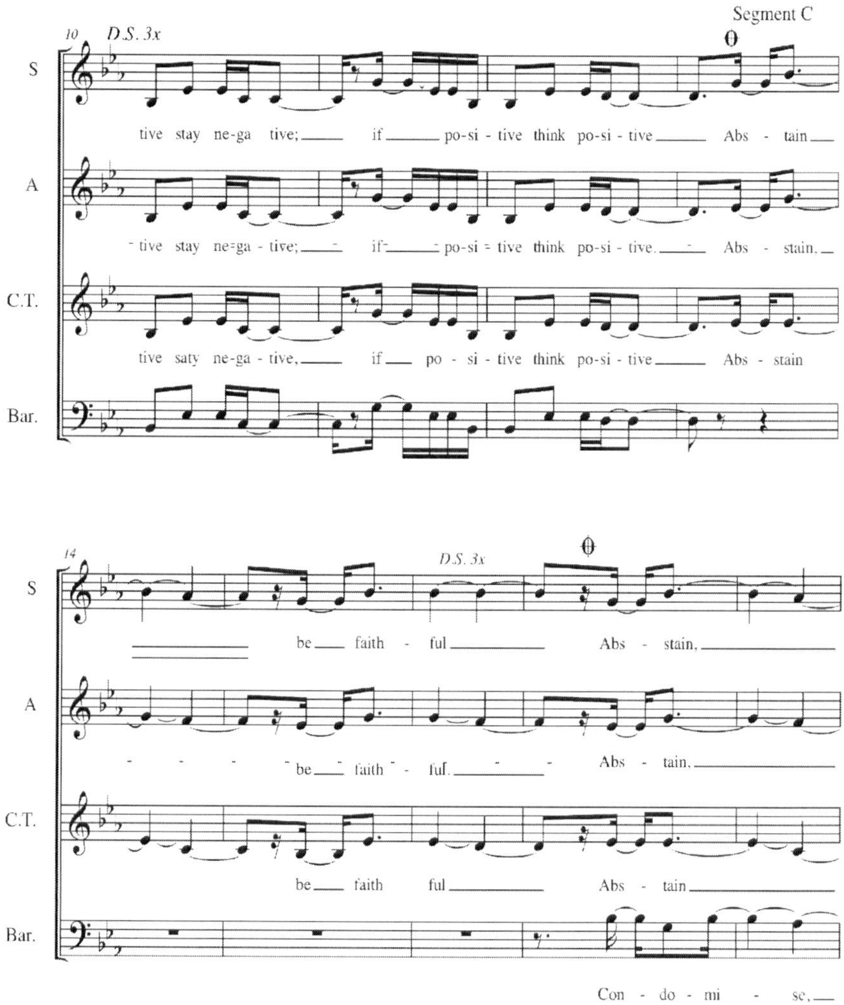
Segment C
D.S. 3x
S
A
C.T.
Bar.
tive stay ne-ga tive; if po-si - tive think po-si - tive Abs - tain
tive stay ne-ga - tive; if po-si - tive think po-si - tive. Abs - stain,
tive saty ne-ga - tive, if po - si - tive think po-si - tive Abs - stain
be faith - ful Abs - stain,
be faith - ful. Abs - tain,
be faith ful Abs - tain
Con - do - mi - se,

3 **YOU'VE GOT TO KNOW YOUR STATUS**

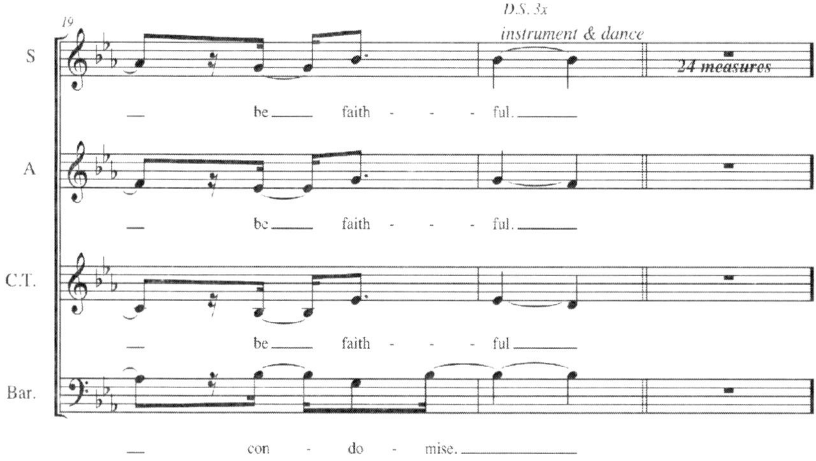

19
D.S. 3x
instrument & dance
24 measures
S
— be faith - - - ful.
A
— be faith - - - ful.
C.T.
— be faith - - - ful
Bar.
— con - do - mise.

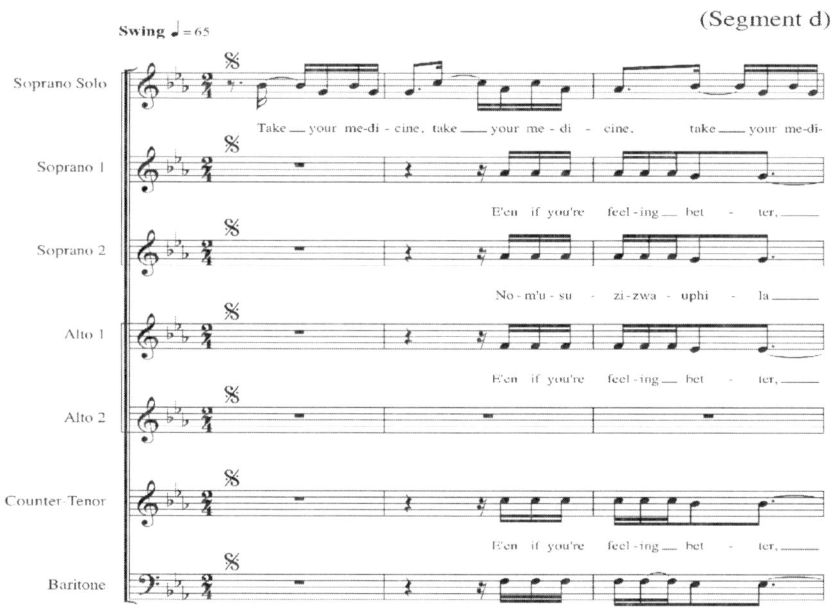

(Segment d)
Swing ♩ = 65
Soprano Solo
Take your me-di - cine, take your me - di - cine, take your me-di-
Soprano 1
E'en if you're feel - ing bet - ter,
Soprano 2
No - m'u - su - zi - zwa - uphi - la
Alto 1
E'en if you're feel - ing bet - ter,
Alto 2
Counter-Tenor
E'en if you're feel - ing bet - ter,
Baritone

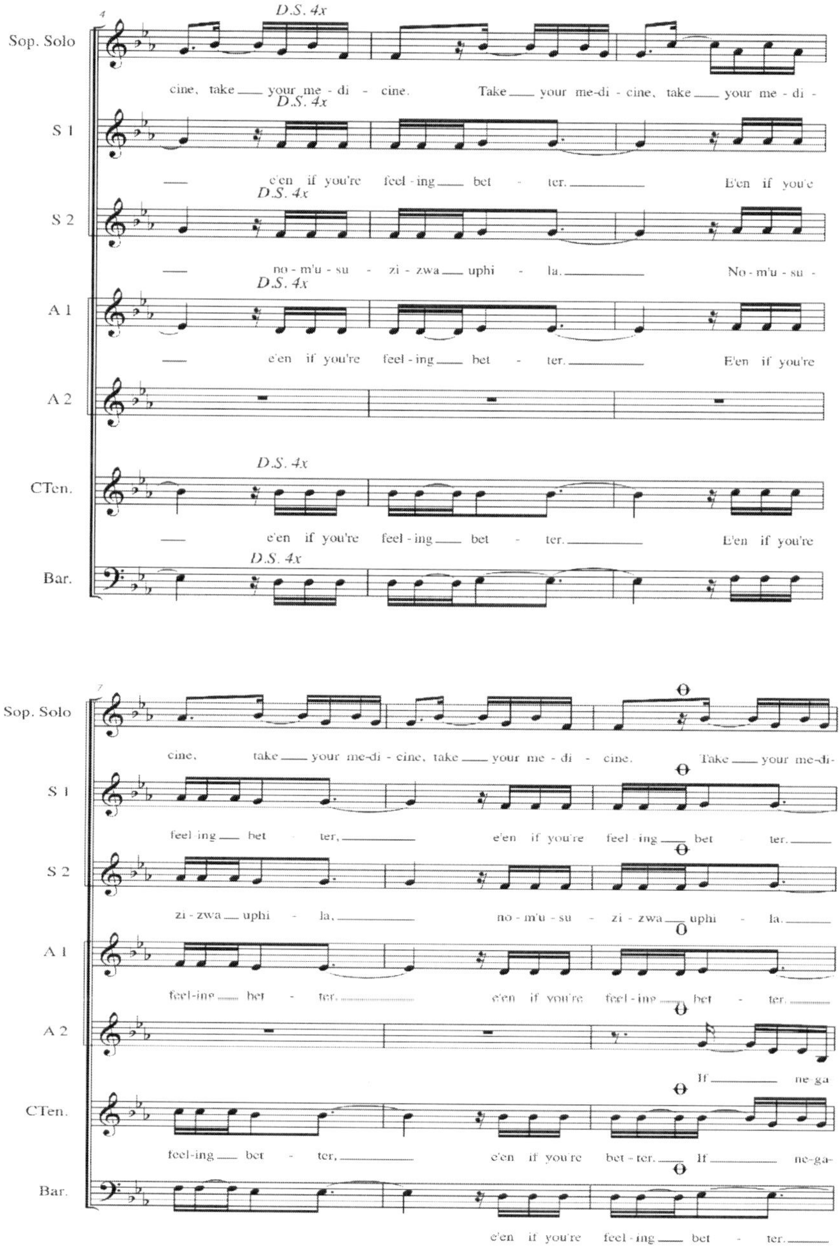
D.S. 4x
Sop. Solo
cine, take your me - di - cine. Take your me-di - cine, take your me - di -
S 1
e'en if you're feel - ing bet - ter. E'en if you'e
S 2
no - m'u - su - zi - zwa uphi - la. No - m'u - su -
A 1
e'en if you're feel - ing bet - ter. E'en if you're
A 2
CTen.
e'en if you're feel - ing bet - ter. E'en if you're
Bar.
Sop. Solo
cine, take your me-di - cine, take your me - di - cine. Take your me-di-
S 1
feel-ing bet - ter, e'en if you're feel - ing bet - ter.
S 2
zi - zwa uphi - la, no - m'u - su - zi - zwa uphi - la.
A 1
feel-ing bet - ter. e'en if you're feel - ing bet - ter.
A 2
If ne-ga
CTen.
feel-ing bet - ter, e'en if you're bet - ter. If ne-ga-
Bar.
e'en if you're feel - ing bet - ter.

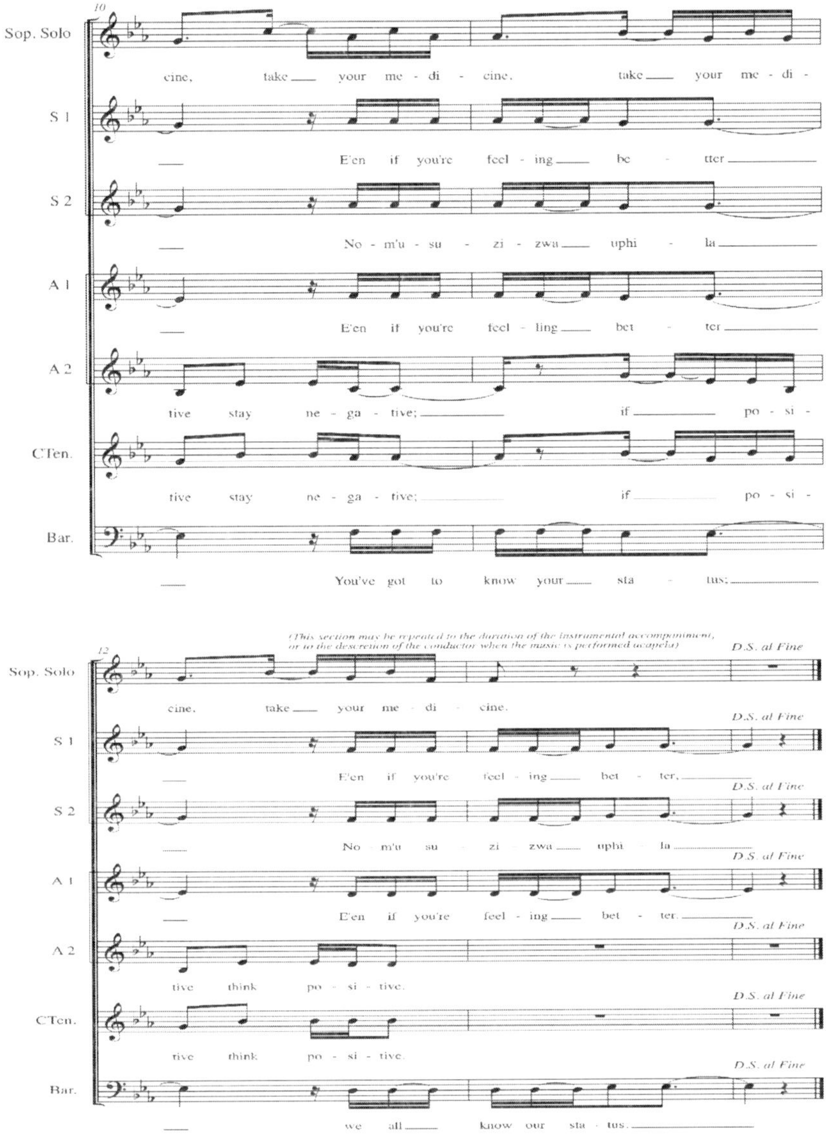
10
Sop. Solo
cine, take your me - di - cine, take your me - di -
S 1
E'en if you're feel - ing be - tter
S 2
No - m'u - su - zi - zwa uphi - la
A 1
E'en if you're feel - ling bet - ter
A 2
tive stay ne - ga - tive; if po - si -
CTen.
tive stay ne - ga - tive; if po - si -
Bar.
You've got to know your sta - tus;
(This section may be repeated to the duration of the instrumental accompaniment, or to the descretion of the conductor when the music is performed acapela)
D.S. al Fine
12
Sop. Solo
cine, take your me - di - cine.
S 1
E'en if you're feel - ing bet - ter,
S 2
No m'u su zi zwa uphi la
A 1
E'en if you're feel - ing bet - ter.
A 2
tive think po - si - tive.
CTen.
tive think po - si - tive.
Bar.
we all know our sta - tus.

Bibliography

Abu-Lughod, Lila. 1993. *Writing Women's Worlds: Bedouin Stories*. Berkeley: University of California Press.

Adelzadeh, Asghar. 2003. "The Challenge of Sustainable Development: Unlocking People's Creativity." In *South African Human Development Report 2003*. Cape Town: UNDP, 2003.

Allwood, Clifford. 1989. "Mission as Healing the Sick: Christian Medical Mission in South Africa." *Missionalia* 7(2): 123–124.

"AM Live." *SAFM 105.1*. 2007. Johannesburg, South Africa: SABC.

Amin, Samir. 2006. *Beyond US Hegemony? Assessing the Prospects for a Multipolar World*. Durban: South Africa: UKZN Press.

Appiah, Kwame A. 1992. *In My Father's House: Africa in the Philosophy of Culture*. New York: Oxford University Press.

ARHAP. 2006. "Appreciating Access: The Contribution of Religion to Universal Access in Africa." *Journal of Theology for Southern Africa* 12(126): 120–126.

Axelsson, Olof E. 1974. "Historical Notes on Neo-African Church Music." *Zambezia: Journal of the University of Rhodesia* 3(2): 89–102.

Barber, Karin.1997. "Introduction." In *Readings in African Popular Culture*, edited by Karin Barber, 1–12. Oxford: James Currey.

Barz, Gregory. 2006. *Singing for Life: HIV/AIDS and Music in Uganda*. New York: Routledge.

Barz, Gregory and Judah Cohen. 2008. "Music and HIV/AIDS in Africa." In *The Garland Handbook of African Music*, edited by Ruth M. Stone, 148–159. New York and London: Routledge, Taylor and Francis Group.

____. 2011. *The Culture of AIDS in Africa: Hope and Healing Through Music and the Arts*. London and New York: Oxford University Press.

Battle, Michael. 1997. *Reconciliation: The Ubuntu Theology of Desmond Tutu*. Cleveland, Ohio: The Pilgrim Press.

Baum, Dan. 2003. "Jake Leg: How the Blues Diagnosed a Medical Mystery." *New Yorker, Annals of Epidemiology*. http://archives.newyorker.com/global/print.asp cited on 01/20/2014.

Bauman, Richard. 2001. "Genre." In *Key Terms in Language and Culture*, edited by Alessandro Duranti. Cambridge: Blackwell.

Baxen, Jean and Breidlid, Anders. Eds. 2009. *HIV/AIDS in Sub-Saharan Africa: Understanding the Implications of Culture and Context.* Singapore: United Nations University Press.

Bebey, Francis. 1975. *African Music: A People's Art.* New York: L. Hills.

Berglund, Axel-Ivar. 1989. *Zulu Thought-Patterns and Symbolism.* Bloomington and Indianapolis: Indiana University Press.

Byerly, Ingrid. 1998. Mirror, Mediator, and Prophet: The Music Indaba of Late -Apartheid South Africa. *Ethnomusicology* 42(1): 1–44.

Biko, Steve. 1971. "Some African Cultural Concepts." In *I Write What I Like -Steve Biko: A Selection of His Writings.* Edited by Aelred C. R. Stubbs [2004], 44–51. Johannesburg: Picador Africa.

———. 1972. "White Racism and Black Consciousness." In *I Write What I Like -Steve Biko: A Selection of His Writings.* Edited by Aelred C. R. Stubbs [2004], 66–79. Johannesburg: Picador Africa.

Blacking, John. 1973. *How Musical Is Man?* Seattle: University of Washington Press.

———. 1995. "The Music of Politics." In *Music, Culture, and Experience*, edited by Reginald Byron, 199–222. Chicago: University of Chicago Press.

Bokwe, John Knox. 1885. *Amaculo aseLovedale.* Eastern Cape, South Africa: Lovedale Institution Press.

Booth, Karen M. 2004. *Local Women, Global Science: Fighting AIDS in Kenya.* Bloomington and Indianapolis: Indiana University Press.

Bornman, Elirea. 2006. "National symbols and nation-building in the post-apartheid South Africa." *International Journal of Intercultural Relations* 30(3): 383–399. *Boston Globe.* February 17, 2003.

Bourgault, Louise M. 2003. *Playing for Life: Performance in Africa in the Age of AIDS.* Durham, North Carolina: Carolina Academic Press.

Boustany, Nora. 2006. "AIDS Crisis Shapes Bishop's Stance." *Washington Post,* 26 April.

Briggs, Charles L., and Richard Bauman. 1992. "Genre, Intertextuality, and Social Power." *Journal of Linguistic Anthropology* 2(2): 131–172.

Brummer, Daan. 2002. *Labour Migration and HIV/AIDS in Southern Africa.* Pretoria: International Organization for Migration (Regional Office for Southern Africa).

Burnim, Mellonee V. 1985a. "Black Gospel Music Tradition: A Complex of Ideology, Aesthetic, and Behavior." In *More Than Dancing: Essays on Afro-American Music and Musicians,* edited by Irene V. Jackson, 147–167. Westport, Connecticut: Greenwood Press.

———. 1985b. "Culture Bearer and Tradition Bearer: An Ethnomusicologist's Research on Gospel Music." *Ethnomusicology* 29(3): 432–447.

———. 2001. "Religious Music." In *The United States and Canada,* edited by Ellen Koskoff, 624–636. Garland Encyclopedia of World Music, 3. New York: Garland Publishing.

———. 2006. "Religious Music." In *African American Music: An Introduction*, edited by Mellonee Burnim and Portia Maultsby, 51–77. New York: Routledge.

Byrnes, Rita M. (1996). *South Africa: A Country Study*. Washington: GPO for the Library of Congress. http://countrystudies.us/south-africa/.

Caluza, Reuben T. 1995 (1930). *Caluza's Double Quartet* [CD Recording]. London: Heritage Music Label.

Campbell, Catherine. 1997. "Migrancy, Masculine Identities and AIDS: The Psychosocial Context of HIV Transmission in the South African Gold Mines." *Social Science and Medicine* 45(2): 273–281.

———. 2000. "Selling Sex in the Time of AIDS: The Psychosocial Context of Condom Use by Sex Workers in a Southern African Mine." *Social Science and Medicine* 50: 479–494.

———. 2003. *Letting Them Die: Why HIV/AIDS Prevention Programmes Fail.* Bloomington and Indianapolis: Indiana University Press.

Campbell, Catherine and Williams, Brian. 1999. "Beyond the Biomedical and the Behavioral: Towards an Integrated approach to HIV Prevention in the Southern African Mining Industry." *Social Science and Medicine* 48: 1625–1639.

Canon, Sheri. 2008. "Not a Band Aid: Ghanaian Afro Roots Musician Rocky Dawuni Empowers Locals with his Musical Activism." *Ethnographic Advocacy and the Performance of Public Health in Africa.* Wesleyan University, Middlebury, CT [Unpublished SEM Conference Paper].

Carswell, Wilson J. 1991. "AIDS in Africa and AIDS in South Africa." In *Religious Workshop on HIV/AIDS*. Pretoria: HSRC.

Carton, Benedict. 2003. "The Forgotten Compass of Death: Apocalypse Then and Now in the Social History of South Africa." *Journal of Social History* 37(1): 199–218.

Chaudhuri, Soma. 2012. "Women as Easy Scapegoats: Witchcraft Accusations and Women as Targets in Tea Plantations of India." *Violence Against Women* 8(10), 1213–1234.

Chase, Gilbert. 1992. *America's Music: From the Pilgrims to the Present.* Urbana University of Illinois Press.

Chernoff, John. 1979. *African Rhythms and African Sensibilities: Aesthetics and Social Action in African Musical Idioms.* Chicago and London. The University of Chicago Press.

Chikwem, John O., Chikwem, Susan D., and Louden, Delroy. 2003. *HIV/AIDS/STI Factsbook.* Oxford, PA: Lincoln University.

Chinweizu. 1987. *The West and the Rest of Us: White Predators, Black Slavers, and the African Elite.* Lagos, Nigeria: Pero Press.

Chitnis, Amit, Diana Rawls, and Jim Moore. 2000. "Origin of HIV Type 1 in Colonial French Equatorial Africa?" *AIDS Research and Human Retroviruses* 16(1): 5–8.

Christian Express. 1918. 48 (600): 84–87.

Clarke, Michael. 1975. "Survival in the Field: Implications of Personal Experience in Field Work." *Theory and Society* 2: 95–123.

Cochraine, James. 2006. "Of Bodies, Barriers, Boundaries and Bridges: Ecclesial Practice in the Face of HIV and AIDS." *Journal of Theology for Southern Africa* 2(126): 7–26.

Cockrell, Dale. 1987. "Of Gospel Hymns, Minstrel Shows, and Jubilee Singers: Toward Some Black South African Musics." *American Music* (winter): 417–432.

Comaroff, Jean and John Comaroff. 1986. "Christianity and Colonialism in South Africa." *American Ethnologist* 13(1): 1–22.

Cone, James. 1969. *Black Theology and Black Power*. New York: Seabury Press.

Coplan, David B. 1985. *In Township Tonight: South Africa's Black City Music and Theatre*. Johannesburg: Ravan Press.

———. 1987. "Eloquent Knowledge: Lesotho Migrants! Songs and the Anthropology of Experience." *American Ethnologist* 14(3): 413–433.

Crichton, J. D. 1980. *Praying and Singing*. London: Collins Liturgical Publications.

Crombie, John W. 1890 (1891). *Some Poets of the People in Foreign Lands*. London: Eliot Stock.

Crosby, Alfred W. 1976. *Epidemic and Peace, 1918*. Westport, CT: Greenwood Press; Reprinted with a new introduction as *America's Forgotten Pandemic: The Influenza of 1918*. New York and London: Cambridge University Press, 1989.

Cross, Wilbur. 2008. "Gullah Culture in America." Westport, Connecticut: Praeger.

Crowe, Barbara J. 2004. *Music and Soulmaking: Toward a New Theory of Music Therapy*. Lanham, MD: Scarecrow Press.

Danielson, Virginia. 1997. *"The Voice of Egypt": Umm Kulthum, Arabic Song, and Egyptian Society in the Twentieth Century*. Chicago: University of Chicago Press.

Dargie, David. 1997. "Christian Music among Africans." In *Christianity in South Africa: A Political, Social, and Cultural History*, edited by Richard Elphick and Rodney Davenport, 319–326. Cape Town: David Philip.

Davenport, Thomas R. H. 1987. *South Africa: A Modern History*. Toronto, Canada: University of Toronto Press.

Day, Dick. 2003. "Preventing HIV/AIDS Via Biblically Based Concepts of Sexuality, Love, and Marriage." In *The Hope Factor: Engaging the Church in the HIV/AIDS Crisis*, edited by David Dageforde, Tetsunao Yamamoriand Tina Bruner, 173–184. Waynesboro, GA: Authentic Media.

de Gruchy, John and de Gruchy, Steve. 2005. *The Church Struggle in South Africa*. Minneapolis: Fortress Press.

DeNoon, Daniel J. 2009. "AIDS in America: Real Patients and Real Doctors Talk to Webmd About the Stigma of HIV, the Medicines, and Hope for the Future." PubMed, http://www.webmd.com/hiv-aids/guide/aids-america.

Derrida, Jacques. 1995. *Archive Fever: A Freudian Impression*. Chicago: University of Chicago Press.

Detterbeck, Markus. 2002. "South African Choral Music (Amakwaya): Song, Contest and the Formation of Identity." Ph.D. dissertation, University of KwaZulu-Natal, Durban.

Diakonia Council of Churches. 2006. *The Oikos Journey: A Theological Reflection on the Economic Crisis in South Africa*. Durban: Diakonia.

Diallo, Yaya Hall Mitchell. 1989. *The Healing Drum: African Wisdom Teachings*. Rochester, VT: Destiny Books.

DiClemente, R. J., and Wingwood, G. M. 1995. "A Randomized Controlled Trial of an HIV Sexual Risk-Education Intervention for Young African American Women." *JAMA* 274: 1271–1276.

Dorrington, Rob, Leigh Johnson, Debbie Bradshor, and Timothy-John Daniel. 2006. *The Demographic Impact of HIV/AIDS in South Africa: National and Provincial*

Indicators for 2006. Cape Town: The Medical Research Council and the Center for Actuarial Research.

Dowden, Richard. 2009. *Africa: Altered States, Ordinary Miracles*. London: Portobello Books Ltd.

Duran, Lucy. 1989. "Key to N'Dour: Roots of the Senegalese Star." *Popular Music* 8(3): 275–84.

Edgar, Robert R., and Hilary Sapire. 2000. "African Apocalypse: The Story of Nontetha Nkwenkwe, a Twentieth-Century South African Prophet." Johannesburg: Witwatersrand University Press.

Eiselen, W. W. M. 1948. "The Meaning of Apartheid." *Race Relations* 15(3): 69–86.

Elia, Nada. 2001. *Trances, Dances, and Vociferations: Agency and Resistance in Africana Women's Narratives*. New York: Garland Publishing.

Elphick, Richard. 1997. "The Benevolent Empire and the Social Gospel: Missionaries and South African Christians in the Age of Segregation." In *Christianity in South Africa: A Political, Social and Cultural History*, edited by Richard Elphick and Rodney Davenport, 347–369. Los Angeles: University of California Press.

Emerson, Robert M., Rachel I. Fretz, and Linda L. Shaw. 1995. *Writing Ethnography*. Chicago: University of Chicago Press.

Emoff, Ron. 2001. *Recollecting from the Past: Musical Practice and Spirit Possession on the East Coast of Madagascar*. Middletown, CT: Wesleyan University Press.

———. 2002. "Maresaka and the Value in Things: Tromba Spirit Possession on the East Coast of Madagascar." In *The Interrelatedness of Music, Religion, and Ritual in African Performance Practice*, edited by Danile K. Avorgbedor, 129–151. Lewiston, NY: Edwin Mellen Press.

Erlmann, Veit. 1990. "Migration and Performance: Zulu Migrant Workers' Isicathamiya Performance in South Africa, 1890–1950." *Ethnomusicology* 34(2): 199–220.

———. 1991. *African Stars: Studies in Black South African Performance*. Chicago: University of Chicago Press.

———. 1995. Reuben Caluza and His Double Quartet [CD Liner Note], London: HMV Records (1930), Re-mastered and re-released by Heritage Music label (1995).

———. 1996. *Nightsong: Performance, Power, and Practice in South Africa*. Chicago: University of Chicago Press.

Etherington, Norman. 1997. "Kingdoms of This World and the Next: Christian Beginnings among Zulu and Swazi." In *Christianity in South Africa: A Political, Social, and Cultural History*, edited by Richard Elphick and Rodney Davenport, 89–106. Los Angeles: University of California Press.

———. 2002. "Outward and Visible Signs of Conversion in Nineteenth-Century Kwazulu-Natal." *Journal of Religion in Africa* 32(4): 422–439.

Farmer, Paul. 1997. "On Suffering and Structural Violence: A View from Below." In *Social Suffering*, edited by Arthur Kleiman, Veena Das, and Margaret Lock, 261–283. Berkeley: University of California Press.

———. 1999. *Infections and Inequalities: The Modern Plagues*. Berkeley: University of California Press.

———. 2003. *Pathologies of Power*. Berkeley: University of California Press.

Fassin, Didier. 2007. *When Bodies Remember: Experience and Politics of AIDS in South Africa*. Berkeley: University of California Press.

Feld, Steven. 1982. *Sound and Sentiment: Birds, Weeping, Poetics, and Song in Kaluli Expression*. Philadelphia: University of Pennsylvania Press.

Feldman, Allen. 1994. "On Cultural Anesthesia: From Desert Storm to Rodney King." *American Ethnologist* 21(2): 404–418.

Fenner, Frank, Henderson, Donald A., Arita, Isao, Ježek, Zdeněk, and Ladnyi, Ivan D. 1988. *Smallpox and Its Eradication*. Geneva: World Health Organization.

Floyd, Samuel A. 1995. *The Power of Black Music: Interpreting Its History from Africa to the United States*. London and New York: Oxford University Press.

"Focus on Senegal." *Roll Back Malaria, Progress and Impact Series Report,* World Health Organization, No. 4, 16–20.

Foucault, Michel. 1980. *Power and Knowledge*. Brighton: Harvester.

Freund, Bill, and Vishnu Padayachee. 1998. "Post-Apartheid South Africa: The Key Patterns Emerge" *Economic and Political Weekly* 33(20): 1173–1180.

Friedson, Steven M. 1996. *Dancing Prophets: Musical Experience in Tumbuka Healing*. Chicago: University of Chicago Press.

———. 2002. "The Disease of the Prophets: The Musical Construction of Clinical Reality." In *The Interrelatedness of Music, Religion, and Ritual in African Performance Practice*, edited by Daniel K Avorgbedor, 155–189. Lewiston, N.Y.: Edwin Mellen Press.

Gaynor, Mitchell L. 1999. *Sounds of Healing: A Physician Reveals the Therapeutic Power of Sound, Voice, and Music*. New York: Broadway Books.

Germond, Paul, and Sepetla Molapo. 2006. "In Search of Bophelo in a Time of Aids: Seeking a Coherence of Economies of Health and Economies of Salvation." *Journal of Theology for Southern Africa* 2(126): 27–47.

Gevisser, Mark. 2001. "AIDS: The New Apartheid." In *The Nation*. http://www.thenation.com/article/aids-new-apartheid/ (accessed on October 20, 2014).

Ghebo, Philip. 1954. "Letter to the Editor." *AMS Newsletter* 1(1): 80–83.

Gilbert, Leah, and Liz Walker. 2002. "HIV/AIDS in South Africa: An Overview." *Cadernos de Saude Publica* 18(3): 651–660.

Gilbert, M. Thomas P., Andrew Rambaut, Gabriela Wlasiuk, Thomas J. Spira, Arthur E. Pitchenik, and Michael Worobey. 2007. "The Emergence of HIV/AIDS in the Americas and Beyond." *Proceedings of the National Academy of Sciences of the United States of America* 104 (47): 18566–18570.

Goba, Bonganjalo. 1974. "Corporate Personality: Ancient Israel and Africa." In *The Challenge of Black Theology,* B. Moore ed. Atlanta, GA: John Knox.

Goffman, Erving. 1989. "On Fieldwork." *Journal of Contemporary Ethnography* 18: 123–132.

"Gospel Queen, Inspirational Role Model: Rebecca Malope." N.d. *South African Music Rights Organization*. http://www.samro.org.za/index.pl (accessed 1 March 2009).

Gottlieb, Alma. 1990. "Hot Blood, Vengeful Blood: AIDS and Blood Symbolism in Africa." In *The Impact of AIDS on Maternal-Child Health Care Delivery in Africa*. Urban: University of Illinois at Urbana-Champaign.

———. 1992. *Under the Kapok Tree: Indentity and Difference in Beng Thought*. Chicago and London: University of Chicago Press.

Gouk, Penelope. 2000. *Musical Healing in Cultural Contexts*. Aldershot: Brookfield.

Greenstein, Ran. 2009. "Alternative Modernity: Development Discourse in Post-apartheid South Africa." *International Social Science Journal* 60(195): 69–84.

Gutierrez, Gustavo. 1973. *A Theology of Liberation: History, Politics, and Salvation.* Maryknoll, New York: Orbis Books

Hainsworth, Sahwn. 2005. *Raising Their Voices: The Sinikithemba Choir.* Philadelphia. Video documentary.

Hall, Stuart. 2003. "The Work of Representation." In *Representation: Cultural Representations and Signifying Practices,* edited by Stuart Hall, 13–76. London: Sage Publications.

Hamm, Charles. 1988. *Afro-American Music, South Africa, and Apartheid.* New York: Institute for Studies in America Music.

Hansen, Deidre Doris. 1968. *The Life and Work of Benjamine Tyamshe: A Contemporary Xhosa Composer.* Grahamstown: Rhodes University.

Henderson, Clara. 1995. "A Paradigm of Africanization: Music of Mvano Women of the Church of Central Africa Presbyterian, Malawi." Master's thesis, Indiana University.

Hildi Hendrickson, ed. *Clothing and Difference: Embodied Identities in Colonial and Post-Colonial Africa.* Duke University Press, 1996.

Hirsch, Lee. 2002. *Amandla: A Revolution in Four-Part Harmony.* DVD. Santa Monica, CA: Artisan.

"HIV in the United States: *At A Glance." Center for Disease Control.* http://www.cdc.gov/hiv/statistics/basics/ataglance.html (accessed November 28, 2014).

HIV & AIDS And STI Strategic Plan For South Africa, 2007–2011. *HIV Surveillance Supplemental Report* 2014, 19(3). Published November 2014.

Hodgson, Janet. 1980. *Ntsikana's Great Hymn: A Xhhosa Expression of Christianity in the Early 19th Century Eastern Cape.* Communications, 4. Rondebosch, South Africa: University of Cape Town Press.

Hopkins, Donald R. 2002. *Smallpox: The Greatest Killer in History.* Chicago: University of Chicago Press.

Howden, John. 2009. "Pfizer to pay £50m after deaths of Nigerian children in drug trial experiment. Out of court settlement in the case that inspired 'The Constant Gardener'." *The Independent World,* 20 April. http://www.independent.co.uk/news/world/africa (accessed 5 April 2010).

Hunt. C. W. 1989. "Migrant labor and sexually transmitted disease: AIDS in Africa." *Journal of Health and Social Behavior* 30(4): 353–73.

———. 1996. "Social Vs Biological: Theories on the Transmission of AIDS in Africa." *Social Science and Medicine* 42(9): 1283–1296.

Hunter, Mark. 2007. "The Changing Political Economy of Sex in South Africa: The Significance of Unemployment and Inequalities to the Scale of the AIDS Pandemic." *Social Science & Medicine* 64(3): 689–700.

Hurley, Denis. N.d. *History of Diakonia.* http://www.diakonia.org.za/ (accessed 25 March 2008).

Hutcheon, Linda. 1985. *A Theory of Parody: The Teachings of Twentieth-Century Art Forms.* New York: Methuen.

Hutcheon, Linda and Hutcheon, Michael. 1996. *Opera: Desire, Disease, Death.* Lincoln and London: University of Nebraska Press.

Jabavu, John T. 1890. *Imvo Zabantsundu*, 16 October.

Janis, Tim. 2002. *A Thousand Summers: Special Aids in Africa Benefit Edition*. CD liner note. Boston, MA: Church World Service.

Jochelson, K., M. Mothiebile, and J. Leger. 1991. "Human Immunodeficiency Virus and Migran Labor in South Africa." *International Journal of Health Services* 21(1): 157–173.

John L. Dube: A Biographical Sketch. N.d. http://www.oberlin.edu/external/EOG/Dube/Dube.htm (accessed 15 September 2009).

Johnson, Mark. 1987. *The Body in the Mind: The Bodily Basis of Meaning, Imagination and Reason*. Chicago: University of Chicago Press.

Johnson, Niall P. A. S., and Mueller, Jurgen. 2002. "Updating the Accounts: Global Mortality of the 1918–1920 "Spanish" Influenza Pandemic." *Bulletin of the History of Medicine* 76: 105–115.

Kaemmer, John E. 1967. "African music and its Significance for the Divine Service," in *Report on the Consultation of African Church Music held by the Christian Academy at Roodekrans*, December 1967, Johannesburg, Christian Academy in Southern Africa.

———. 2008. "Southern Africa: An Introduction." In *The Garland Handbook of African Music*. Ruth M. Stone ed. 382–405 (Second Edition), New York and London: Routledge, Taylor & Francis Group.

Kani, John. 2002. *Nothing but the Truth*. Johannesburg: Witswatersrand University Press.

Kauffman, Kyle D. 2004. "Why Is South Africa the HIV Capital of the World? An Institutional Analysis of the Spread of a Virus." In *AIDS and South Africa: The Social Expression of a Pandemic*, edited by Kyle D. Kauffman and David L. Lindauer, 17–30. New York: Palgrave Macmillan.

Keteyi, Xolile S. J. 1998. *Inculturation as a Strategy for Liberation: A Challenge for South Africa*. Pietermaritzburg: Cluster Publications.

Kirby, Percival R. 1937. "Saint Cecilia Goes South: A Contribution to the History of Music in South Africa." *Paper presented at the Proceedings of the Musical Association, 64th session*. London: Oxford University Press.

Kivnick, Helen Q. 1990. *Where Is the Way: Song and Struggle in South Africa*. New York: Penguin Books.

Koen, Benjamin D. 2003. "Devotional Music and Healing in Badakhstan, Tajikistan: Preventive and Curative Practices." Ph.D. Dissertation, Ohio State University.

———. 2006. "Musical Healing in Eastern Tajikistan: Transforming Stress and Depression through Falak Performance." *Asian Music* 37(2): 58–83.

Kopelman, Loretta M. 2002. "If HIV/AIDS is Punishment, Who is Bad?" *The Journal of Medicine and Philosophy* 27(2): 231–243.

Krige, Jensen E. 1950. *The Social System of the Zulus*. Pietermaritzburg: Shuter & Shooter.

KZN. N.d. "Royal Reed Dance 2006 Press Release." www.kzn.org.za/kzn/news/ (accessed 23 September 2008).

Lane, Deforia, and Rob Wilkins. 1994. *Music as Medicine: Deforia Lane's Life of Music, Healing, and Faith*. Grand Rapids, MI: Zondervan.

Langford, Christopher. 2002. "The Age Pattern of Mortality in the 1918–19 Influenza Pandemic: An Attempted Explanation Based on Data for England and Wales." *Medical History* 46: 1–20.

L'Abbe, E. N. Henderson, Z. L., and Loots, M. 2003. "Uncovering a Nineteenth-Century Typhoid Epidemic at the Koffiefontein Mine, South Africa." *World Archeology [Archaeology of Epidemic and Infectious Disease]* 35(2): 306–318.

Latta, Judi M. 1999. "'Wade in the Water,' the Public Radio Series: The Effects of the Politics of Production on Sacred Music Representations." Ph.D. dissertation, University of Maryland.

Le Baron, Curt. 2006. "Microethnography." *The SAGE Dictionary of Social Research Methods.* Victor Jupp, ed. London: SAGE Publications Ltd.

Lingerman, Hal A. 1995. *The Healing Energies of Music.* 2nd ed. Wheaton, IL: Theosophical Publishing House.

L. M. P. 1870s. "Service in a Native Chapel." In *American Zulu Mission: Extracts from the Journal Life and Light for Woman*, 337. Durban: Killi Campbell Africana Library.

Lwanda, John. 2003. "Orality Music and HIV/AIDS: Interrogating the Malawi Popular Public Sphere." *Africa on a Global Stage—Australasia and the Pacific African Studies Association, Australasia and the Pacific.* 1–20.

Machen, Peter. N.d. *Marianhill Monastery, Ethekwini Municipality.* www.durban.gov.za/durban/discover-durban (accessed 26 September 2008).

Magaziner, Daniel. 2010. *The Law and the Prophets: Black Consciousness in South Africa, 1968–1977.* Athens: Ohio University Press.

Magkoba, Sindiwe. 2007. *Personal Conversation.* Hillcrest, KwaZulu-Natal, South Africa, 15 March, 2007.

Maultsby, Porta K. 2005. "Africanisms in African American Music." In *Africanisms in American Culture*, edited by Joseph E. Holloway, 326–355. Bloomington: Indiana University Press.

Mbembe, Achille. 2002. "African Modes of Self-Writing." *Public Culture* 14(1): 239–273.

Mbiti. 1970. *African Religions and Philosophy.* London: Doubleday Books.

McCall, John C. 2000. *Dancing Hisotries: Heuristic Ethnography with the Ohafia Igbo.* Ann Arbor: University of Michigan Press.

McCord, James B., and Douglas, John Scott. 1946. *My Patients were Zulus.* New York and Toronto: Rinehart and Co., Inc.

McCord, Margaret. 2000. *The Calling of Katie Makanya.* Johannesburg: David Philip.

Meadows, Peter. 2003. "A Letter to the U.K. Church." In *The Hope Factor: Engaging the Church in the HIV/AIDS Crisis*, edited by David Dageforde, Tetsunao Yamamori, and Tina Bruner, 147–156. Waynesboro, GA: Authentic Publication.

Meintjes, Louise, 2003. Sound of Africa: *Making Music Zulu in a South African Studio.* Durham, SC: Duke University Press.

Mercer, Kobena. 1990. "Traveling Theory: The Cultural Politics of Race and Representation." *Afterimage*, interview by Lorraine Kenny, 18: 7–9.

Meriam, Alan. 1967. "The Use of Music as a Technique of Reconstructing Culture History in Africa." In *Reconstructing African Culture History,* edited by Creighton Gavel and Norman R. Benett, 85–114. Boston: Boston University Press.

Muller, Carol A. 2002. "Archiving Africanness in Sacred Song." *Ethnomusicology* 46(3): 409–31.

———. 2004. *South African Music: A Century of Traditions in Transformation.* Santa Barbara, CA: ABC CLIO.

Murren, Keefe, and Walker, Nelson. 2004. *Ithemba-Hope*. Boston: Film Documentary.

Myburgh, James. N.d. "The Virodene Affair (V): How the Efficacy of Virodene Was Finally Put to the Test, and Why the War on Anti-Retrovirals Ended." *COSATU Daily News*. http://groups-beta.google.com/group/COSATU-Daily-News (accessed 8 April 2009).

Motshekga, Mathole. 2007. "On Ubuntu." *Afternoon Show with Xolani Gwala, SAFM 105.1*. Johannesburg, South Africa: SABC.

"National Finals Programme." 2006. *Old Mutual / Telkom National Choir Festival at the Nelson Mandela Metropolitan University*. Port Elizabeth, South Africa.

Nattrass, Nicoli. 2004. *The Moral Economy of AIDS in South Africa*. Cambridge, MA: Cambridge University Press.

———. 2007. *Mortal Combat: Aids Denialism and the Struggle for Antiretrovirals in South Africa*. Scottsville: University of KwaZulu-Natal Press.

Ndungane, Njongonkulu. 2003. *A World with a Human Face: A Voice from Africa*. Cape Town: David Philip.

Nene, Thokozani. 2006. *Personal Conversation*. Lamonstville, South Africa.

———. 2007. *Personal Conversation*. Lamonstville, South Africa.

Ngema, Mbogeni, and William Nicholson. [1987] 2002. *Sarafina*. DVD. Directed by Darrell Roodt. Performed by Whoopi Goldberg, Leleti Khumalo, Miriam Makeba, and others. Screenplay based on the play by Mbogeni Ngema. Buena Vista Home Entertainment.

Nicholson, Karl G., Robert G. Webster, and Alan J. Hay. 1998. *Textbook of influenza*. Blackwell Science Ltd.

Nketia, J. H. Kwabena. 1974. *The Music of Africa*. New York: W. W. Norton.

Norval, Aletta J.1996. *Deconstructing Apartheid*. London and New York: Verso.

Ntsimane, Radikobo. 2006. "To Disclose or Not to Disclose: An Appraisal of the Memory Box Project as a Safe Space for Disclosure of HIV Positive Status." *Journal of Theology for Southern Africa* 1(125): 7–20.

Obeng, Samuel G. 2003. *Language in African Social Interaction: Indirectness in Akan Communication*. New York: Nova Science Publishers.

Okigbo, Austin C. 2011. "Performing Blackness in a South African HIV/AIDS Choir." *Du Bois Review* 8(1): 241–251.

———. 2014. "Contesting Cultural Meaning in a Post-Apartheid South Africa HIV/AIDS Music Event." *African Music* 9(4): 54–70.

Okigbo, Austin C., and Ezumah, Bellarmine A. 2015. "Media Health Images of Africa and the Politics of Representation: A South African AIDS Choir Counter-Narrative." *Journal of Asian and African Studies*: 0021909615608208.

Old Mutual Music http://dogreatthings.co.za/music/2015-prescribed-music/ [accessed February 14, 2016].

O'Loughlin, Bill. 2008. "Deanna: Exercise Can Transform You." http://napwa.org.au/pl/2008/07/deanna-exercise-can-transform-you (accessed 8 April 2009).

Olwage, Grant. 2008. "Introduction." In *Composing Apartheid: Music for and Against Apartheid*. Grant Olwage, ed. 1–10, Johannesburg: Wits University Press.

———. 2008. "Apartheid's Musical Signs" Reflections on Black Choralism, Modernity and Race-ethnicity in the Segregation Era." In *Composing Apartheid: Music for and Against Apartheid.* Grant Olwage, ed. 35–53, Johannesburg: Wits University Press.

"One South African Bishop Supports Condoms to Prevent AIDS." 2002. In *TRC Report: News and Views from the Religious Consultation on Population, Reproductive Health, and Ethics* 5(2).

PACSA. 2004. "Gender, Poverty and HIV/AIDS: What Ordinary People Living with HIV/AIDS Want Decision Makers to Know." *Newsletter.* Pietermaritzburg: PACSA.

Parker, Beverly. 1997. *The Music Department, Its Options, Its Thinking in Terms of the Future: Interview with South African Broadcasting Corporation.* Durban: SABC.

Parnell, Susan. 1991. "Sanitation, Segregation and the Natives (Urban Areas) Act: African exclusion from Johannesburg's Malay Location, 1897–1925" *Journal of Historical Geography* 17(3): 271–288.

Parrinder, Geofery. 1946. 'Worship in Protestant Missions.' *International Review of Missions* 35(2): 187–193.

Pellman, John. 2006. *Morning Edition with John Pellman.* Radiobroadcast. Johannesburg: SABC.

Pembrey, Graham. N.d. "The Scale of South Africa's AIDS Crisis." www.avert.org/aidssouthafrica.htm (accessed 18 February 2008).

Perham, Margery. 1974. *African Apprenticeship: An Autobiographical Journey in Southern Africa, 1929.* London: Faber & Faber.

Phillips, Howard. 1990. *Black October: The Impact of the Spanish Influenza Epidemic of 1918 on South Africa.* Pretoria: Government Printer.

Pietermaritzburg Agency for Christian Social Awareness. 2004. *Fact Sheet No. 52.* Pietermaritzburg, South Africa.

Pinkerton, Lady. 1870. "American Zulu Mission: Extracts from the Journal *Life and Light for Women.*" MS in Killi Campbell African Library, University of KwaZulu-Natal, Durban.

Pittman, K., P. M. Wilson, S. Adams-Taylor, and S. Randolph. 1992. "Making Sexuality Education and Prevention Programs for African American Youth." *Journal of School Health* 62: 339–344.

Plaatje, Solomon. 1921. *Negro World* [editorial], 12 February.

Plan of Action: The Ecumenical Response to HIV/AIDS in Africa. 2001. Nairobi: Global Consultation on the Ecumenical Response to the Challenge of HIV/AIDS in Africa.

Poon, Linda. 2014. "If Salt-N-Pepa Told You To Brush Your Teeth, You'd Surely Listen." *National Public Radio* (NPR Blog). http://www.npr.org/sections/goatsandsoda/2014/08/20/341869218/if-salt-n-pepa-told-you-to-brush-your-teeth-youd-surely-listen (accessed August 24, 2014).

Prejean, Joseph, Ruiguang Song, Angela Hernandez, Rebecca Ziebell, Timothy Green, Frances Walker, and Lillian S. Lin. 2011. "Estimated HIV incidence in the United States, 2006–2009." *PloS one* 6(8): e17502.

"President's 'HIV Cure' Condemned." N.d. *British Broadcasting Corporation.* http://news.bbc.co.uk/2/hi/africa/6323449.stm (accessed 10 April 2009).

Rahfaldt, Michal J. 2007. "Music-Based Radio and Youth Education in South Africa." Ph.D. dissertation, University of Michigan at Ann Arbor.

Ramphele, Mamphela. 2001. "Combating Racism in South Africa: Redress/Remedies." In *Beyond Racism: Race and Inequality in Brazil, South Africa, and the United States*, edited by Charles Hamilton et al., 63–83. Boulder, CO: Lynne Rienner Publishers.

———. 2001. "Citizenship Challenges for South Africa's Young Democracy." *Daedalus* 130(1): 1–17.

Ranger, Terence. 1988. "The Influenza Pandemic in Southern Rhodesia: A Crisis of Comprehension." In Arnold, David, ed. pp. 172–188. *Imperial Medicine and Indigenous Societies*. Manchester, England: Manchester University Press.

Rasmussen, Susan J. 1995. *Spirit Possession and Personhood among the Kel Ewey Tuareg*. Cambridge Studies in Social and Cultural Anthropology. New York, NY: Cambridge University Press.

Roach, Marilynne K. 2013. *Six Women of Salem: The Untold Story of the Accused and Their Accusers in the Salem Witch Trials*. Boston, MA: Da Capo Press.

Reagon, Bernice J. 1992. "Searching for Tindley." In *We'll Understand It Better By and By*, edited by Bernice Johnson Reagon, 37–52. Washington, DC: Smithsonian Institution Press.

Reed, Daniel B. 2003. *Dan Ge Performance: Masks and Music in Contemporary Cote D'Ivoire*. Bloomington: Indiana University Press.

Reese, Gustave. 1959. *Music in the Renaissance*. Rev. ed. New York: W. W. Norton.

Rivière, Philippe. 2002. "In Denial about a Deadly Future: South Africa's AIDS Apartheid." In *Le Monde Diplomatique*. www.http://mondediplo.com/2002/08/04aids (accessed on October 20, 2014).

Robins, Steven. 2004. "'Long Live Zackie, Long Live': AIDS Activism, Science and Citizenship after Apartheid." *Journal of Southern African Studies* 30(3): 651–672.

Rodney, Walter. 1981. *How Europe Underdeveloped Africa*. Washington, DC: Howard University Press.

Rycroft, David K. 1971. "Stylistic Evidence in Nguni Song." In *Essays on Music and History in Africa*, edited by Klaus P. Wachsmann, 213–241. Evanston, IL: Northwestern University Press.

———. 1977. "Evidence of Stylistic Continuity in Zulu Town Music." In *Essays for a Humanist: An Offering to Klaus Wachsmann*, edited by David K. Rycroft, 216–260. Spring Valley, NY: Town House Press.

Samkange, Stanlake J. T., and Tommie M. Samkange. 1980. *Hunhuism or Ubuntuism: A Zimbabawean Indigenous Political Philosophy*. Salisbury: Graham Publications.

Saussure, Ferdinand de. 1960. *Course in General Linguistics*. London: Peter Owen.

Schmid, Barbara. 2006. "AIDS Discourses in the Church: What We Say and What We Do." *Journal of Theology for Southern Africa* 1(125): 91–103. Special edition on HIV/AIDS.

Scorgie, Fiona. 2002. "Virginity Testing and the Politics of Sexual Responsibility: Implications for AIDS Intervention." *African Studies* 61(1): 55–75.

Scully, Nora, and William Charles Scully. 1897. "Kafir Music." *The Pall Mall Magazine*.

Sebidi, Lebamang. 1995. "Interview." In *Sinomlando Project, UKZN Theology Department*. Pietermartizburg: The Alan Paton Center & Struggle Archives.

Sechaba. N.D. "John Langalibalele Dube: First ANC President-General." www.anc.org.za/ancdocs/history/people/dube.html (accessed 2 October 2008).

Seftel, Alan D. 1988. "AIDS and Apartheid: Double Trouble." *African Medical Report* 17–22.

Semouse, Josiah. 1890. *Leselinyana*, 1 October.

Seroff, Doug. 1990. "A Brief Introduction to the Zulu Choirs." *Black Music Research Journal* 10(1): 54–57.

Setiloane, Gabriel. 1973. "Ukubuyisa." *South African Outlook*, 36–41.

Shaffer, Jacqueline. 1956. "Experiments in Indigenous Church Music among the Batetela." *African Music* 1(3): 39–42.

Shelemay, Kay, K. 1997. "The Ethnomusicologist, Ethnographic Method, and the Transmission of Tradition " In *Shadows in the Field: New Perspectives for Fieldwork in Ethnomusicology*, edited by Gregory F. Barz and Timothy J. Cooley, 189–204. New York: Oxford University Press.

Shepherd, Robert H. W. 1941. *Lovedale, South Africa: The Story of a Century, 1841–1941*. Lovedale C. P., South Africa: Lovedale Press.

Sibeko, David M. N.d. *The Sharpeville Massacre: Its Historic Significance in the Struggle against Apartheid.* www.anc.org.za/ancdocs/history/misc/sharplle.html (accessed 22 September 2008).

———. N.d. *Nkosi Sikelel' iAfrika: South Africa's National Anthem.* www.anc.org.za/misc/nkosi.html (accessed 27 November 2008).

Sindima, Harvey J. 1992. *The Legacy of Scottish Missionaries in Malawi.* Studies in the History of Missions, 8. Lewiston, NY: Edwin Mellen Press.

Skoler-Karpoff, S. 2008. "Efficacy of Carraguard for Prevention of HIV Infection in Women in South Africa: A Randomised, Double-Blind, Placebo-Controlled Trial." *Lancet* 372(9654): 1977–1987.

Skota, Mweli T. D. 1931. *The African Yearly Register*. Johannesburg: R. L. Esson & Co.

"Small-Pox In South Africa." *The British Medical Journal* [News Report] 2(1392). 521 (1887).

Smith, Linda T. 1999. *Decolonizing Methodologies: Research and Indigenous Peoples*. London & New York: Zed Books.

"South Africa Marks Key AIDS Milestone." N.d. www.unaids.org (accessed 7 May 2007).

"South African Mayor Defends Virgin Scholarships for Students." http://www.bbc.com/news/world-africa-35403501 (accessed on January 25, 2016).

Southern, Eileen, ed. 1983. *Readings in Black American Music*. New York: W. W. Norton & Company.

Speight, W. L. 1934. "Notes on South African Native Music " *The Musical Quarterly* 20(3): 344–353.

Spindler, Marc R. "Thomas Arbousset, 1810 to 1887, Protestant Lesotho." *Dictionary of African Christian Biography*, http://www.dacb.org/stories/lesotho/arbousset_thomas.html cited on 10/21/2012.

Steingo, Gavin. 2011. "Kwaito and the Culture of AIDS in South Africa." In *The Culture of Aids in Africa: Hope and Healing Through Music and the Arts*. Gregory Barz and Judah Cohen, Eds. 343–61. New York and London: Oxford University Press.

Stephens, Torrence, Ronald L. Braithwaite, and Sandra E. Taylor. 1998. "Model for Using Hip-Hop Music for Small Group HIV/AIDS Prevention Counseling with African American Adolescents and Young Adults." *Patient Education Counseling* 35: 127–137.

Stevenson, H. C., and Davies, G. 1994."Impact of Culturally Sensitive AIDS Video Education on the AIDS Risk Knowledge of African American Adolescents." *AIDS Education Preview* 6: 40–52.

Stoller, Paul. 1989. *Fusion of the Worlds: An Ethnography of Possession Among the Songhay of Niger*. Chicago: University of Chicago Press.

———. 1997. "Globalizing Method: Doing Ethnography in Transnational Spaces." *Anthropology and Humanism* 17(1): 81–95.

Stone, Ruth M. 1982. *Let the Inside Be Sweet: The Interpretation of Music Event among the Kpelle of Liberia*. Bloomington: Indiana University Press.

———. 2005. *Music in West Africa: Experiencing Music, Expressing Culture*. New York: Oxford University Press.

———. 2008. *Theory for Ethnomusicology*. Upper Saddle River, N.J.: Prentice Hall.

Stubbs, Aelred C. R. 2006. "Martyr of Hope: A Personal Memoire." In *Steve Biko: I Write What I Like*, edited by Aelred C. R. Stubbs, 175–244. Johannesburg: Picador Africa.

Sturge, Havelock. 1889. "Notes on an Epidemic of Small-Pox among Kafirs in the Transkei." *The British Medical Journal* 1(1468): 352–353.

Sundkler, Bengt. 1960. *The Christian Ministry in Africa*. Uppsala: Almqvist and Viksells.

The Liber Usualis (1810–1813). 1963. Tournai: Desclée Company.

Theal, George M. 1899. *South Africa*. Cape Colonial Civil Service. 5th Edition; cited in "Small-Pox In The Early Days of Cape Colony," *The British Medical Journal* (1900) 1(2045): 595–596.

Thram, Diane. 2002. "Performance as Ritual, Performance as Art: Therapeutic Efficacy of Dadanda Song and Dance in Zimbabwe." In *The Interrelatedness of Music, Religion, and Ritual in African Performance Practice*, edited by Daniel K. Avorgbedor, 99–125. Lewiston, NY: Edwin Mellen Press.

"Tonic Solfa." N.d. *Encyclopedia Britannica*. www.britannica.com/EBchecked/topic/599276/tonic-solfa (accessed 6 August 2008).

Tracey, Hugh. N.d. *Siwahlula Ngemikhonto*. Grahamstown: ILAM.

Treichler, Paula A. 2004. *How to Have Theory in an Epidemic: Cultural Chronicles of AIDS*. Durham: Duke University Press.

———. 1987. "AIDS, Homophobia, and Biomedical Discourse: An Epidemic of Signification." *AIDS: Cultural Analysis/Cultural Activism* 43(1): 31–70.

Turnbull, Colin M. 1962. *The Lonely African*. New York: Simon & Schuster.

Turner, Victor Witter. 1968. *The Drums of Affliction: A Study of Religious Processes among the Ndembu of Zambia*. Oxford: Clarendon Press; London: International African Institute.

Tutu, Desmond. 1973. "Some African Insights and the Old Testament." In *Relevant Theology for Africa,* edited by Hans-Jurgen Becken, 21–29. Durban: Lutheran Publishing House.

———. 2004. "Preface." In *Steve Biko: I Write What I Like,* edited by Aelred C. R. Stubbs, ix–xiii. Johannesburg: Picador Africa.

"Ubuntu (Philosophy)." 2008. *New World Encyclopedia.* www.newworldencyclopedia.org/entry (accessed 25 February 2010).

UNAIDS. 2006. "Overview of the Global AIDS Epidemic." *Annual Report.* New York: UNAIDS.

UNICEF. 2006. "Africa's Orphaned And Vulnerable Generations Children Affected By AIDS." *Annual Report.* New York: UNICEF.

Van der Vliet, Virginia. 2004. "South Africa Divided Against AIDS: A Crisis of Leadership." In *AIDS and South Africa: The Social Expression of a Pandemic,* edited by Kay Kauffman and D. Lindauer, 48–96. New York: Palgrave Macmillan.

Van Deusen, Kira. 2004. "Singing Story, Healing Drum: Shamans and Storytellers of Turkic Siberia." Montreal: McGill-Queen's University Press.

Vaughan, Peter, Rogers Everett, Arvind M. Singhal, and Ramadhan Swalehe. 2000. "Entertainment-Education and HIV/AIDS Prevention: A Field Experiment in Tanzania." *Journal of Health Communication* 5(suppl.): 81–100.

Viljoen, A. T. 1989. "Apartheid and AIDA." *Lancet* 2: 1280.

Vitillo, Robert J. 1991. "Theology and Transformation: The Challenge of HIV/AIDS to the Church." In *Religious Workshop on HIV/AIDS.* Pretoria: HSRC.

Walker, Adrian. 2003. "Strong Voices for Africa" *Boston Globe,* 17 February, 2003.

"War and Peace." 2003. *Service.* Elkhart, IN: Church World Service, Spring, *Newsletter.*

Waterman, Christopher A. 1990. *Jùjú: A Social History and Ethnography of an African Popular Music.* Chicago: University of Chicago Press.

Wax, Murray L. 1980. "Paradoxes of 'Consent' to the Practice of Fieldwork." *Social Problems* 27: 272–283.

Weman, Henry. 1960. *African Music and the Church in Africa.* Uppsala: Appelbergs Boktryckeri.

Wilson, Olly. 1992. "The Heterogeneous Sound Ideal in African-American Music." In *New Perspectives on Music: Essays in Honor of Eileen Southern.* Eds. Josephine Write and Samuel A. Floyd. Warren, Michigan: Harmonie Park Press.

Wilson, Francis, and Ramphele Mamphela. 1989. *Uprooting Poverty: The South African Challenge: Report for the Second Carnegie Inquiry into Poverty and Development in Southern Africa.* Cape Town: David Philip Publishers.

Wilson, Richard A. 2000. "Reconciliation and Revenge in Post-Apartheid South Africa: Rethinking Legal Pluralism and Human Rights." *Current Anthropology* 41(1): 75–98.

Wolff, David. 1914. *Unter den Sulu: Mancherlei Mitteilungen aus dem Praktischen Missionsdienst.* Hermannsburg: Missionshandlung.

Wood, Barry. 2007. *Personal Conversation.* Durban, South Africa, March 2007.

Worden, Nigel. 1994. *The Making of Modern South Africa: Conquest, Segregation, and Apartheid.* Oxford: Blackwell.

Wylie, Dan. 2006. *Myth of Iron: Shaka in History*. Scottsville: University of KwaZulu-Natal Press.

Xulu, Musa. 1995. "Socio-Political Change and the National Anthem in South Africa: A Critical Appraisal of 'Nkosi Sikelel' Iafrika'." In *Tenth Symposium on Ethnomusicology*. Rhodes University, Grahamstown: ILAM.

Zhu, Tuofu, Bette T. Korber, and Andre J. Nahinias. 1998. "An African HIV-1 Sequence from 1959 and Implications for the Origin of the Epidemic." *Nature* (391): 594–597.

SONGS

Biata, Lihle. 2005. *Ilolo*. [unpublished sol-fa manuscript].

______. 2005. *Inyala*. [unpublished sol-fa manuscript].

Bokwe, John Knox. 1892. "Plea for Africa." In *South Africa Sings* Vol 1. Mzilikazi Khumalo, Editor [1998]. Johannesburg, South Africa: SAMRO.

Caluza, Reuben T. 1919. "Influenza," *Lovedale Sol-fa Leaflets, No. 11c*. Eastern Cape. South Africa. Lovedale Press.

Cleremont Youth Theatre Company. 2007. *The Truth Shall Set You Free* [Unpublished song].*There is a Race that I Must Run. n.d.* [Performed by the South African AIDS Foundation 2005], Glenmore, Durban, South Africa.

"I Feel Pity." In Crombie, John W. 1890 (1891). *Some Poets of the People in Foreign Lands*. London: Eliot Stock.

"Ikhalaphi." n.d. [Zulu folksong, in CD recording with Janis, Tim. 2002. *A Thousand Summers: Special Aids in Africa Benefit Edition*]. Boston, MA: Church World Service.

"Isiyalo." n.d. [Zulu Folkong, performed by Siphithemba Choir], Durban, South Africa: 2007.

Kunene, Phumlani. n.d. *Friendship with Jesus* [recorded with Janis, Tim. 2002. *A Thousand Summers: Special Aids in Africa Benefit Edition*. Boston, MA: Church World Service.

____. n.d. *In Times of Sorrow* [CD recording with Janis, Tim. 2002. *A Thousand Summers: Special Aids in Africa Benefit Edition*]. Boston, MA: Church World Service.

____. n.d. *Know Your Status*. [Unpublished Siphithemba Choir Song].

____. n.d. *Kulukhuni Ezweni*. [CD recording with Janis, Tim. 2002. *A Thousand Summers: Special Aids in Africa Benefit Edition*]. Boston, MA: Church World Service.

____. n.d. *Ngizohamba*. [CD recording with Janis, Tim. 2002. *A Thousand Summers: Special Aids in Africa Benefit Edition*]. Boston, MA: Church World Service.

___. n.d. *Yes, My Lord* [CD recording with Janis, Tim. 2002. *A Thousand Summers: Special Aids in Africa Benefit Edition*]. Boston, MA: Church World Service.

Kunene, Phumlani, and Xolani Zulu. n.d. *Izizwe Mazihloma* [CD recording with Janis, Tim. 2002. *A Thousand Summers: Special Aids in Africa Benefit Edition*]. Boston, MA: Church World Service.

Kunene, Phumlani, Sizwe Ndlela, Zinhle Thabethe, and Xolani Zulu. 2002. *Jehova*. [CD recording with Janis, Tim. 2002. *A Thousand Summers: Special Aids in Africa Benefit Edition*]. Boston, MA: Church World Service.

Kunene, Phumlani and Siphithemba Choir. 1998. *Siyakubonga Somandla* [Unpublished Siphithemba Choir Song].

___. 2003. *Siyaphela Isiwe seNkosi* [Unpublished Siphithemba Choir Song].

Ndlela, Sizwe. 2003. *Sizwile Ukuthi* [Unpublished Siphithemba Choir Song].

"Nkonyane kaNdaba." n.d. [Unpublished folk version, performed by Siphithemba Choir], Durban, 2007.

Shabane, Phakamile. n.d. *Praises.* [Unpublished Song].

Shembe, Isaiah. n.d. *Sindedele Singene.* (Translated by Hugh Tracey, courtesy of the International Library of African Music (ILAM), Rhodes University, Grahamstown, South Africa.

Sontonga, Enoch M. 1941 [1897]. *Nkosi Sikelel' iAfrika.* Lovedale sol-fa leaflets No. 17. Eastern Cape, South Africa: Lovedale Press.

We are Left Outside. n.d. in Crombie, John W. 1890 (1891). *Some Poets of the People in Foreign Lands.* London: Eliot Stock.

We Were Cast Away. n.d. [Buthelezi family song], Hugh Tracey Collection, courtesy of the International Library of African Music (ILAM), Rhodes University, Grahamstown, South Africa.

"Yehla Moya OyiNgcwele." n.d. in *Siyanqoba Ngesiphambano- We Overcome Through the Cross* [Good Friday Ecumenical Service, April 6, 2007], Durban, South Africa: Diakonia Council of Churches.

Index

About the Author

Austin C. Okigbo is assistant professor at the University of Colorado College of Music in Boulder and an affiliate faculty in Ethnic Studies. He received his doctorate in Ethnomusicology and African Studies from Indiana University, Bloomington. His research is on music in African religious experience, diaspora performances, global health, interreligious and inter-cultural dialogues. Okigbo has featured in a number of international radio and television programs including BBC, and Channels TV Lagos as contributor in programs on African music and the entertainment industry. His publications have also appeared in a number of refereed journals including *Africa Today* (Indiana University), *Du Bois Review* (Harvard), and *African Music* (ILAM, South Africa). He is a guest editor of a themed issue of the *World of Music Journal* (Georg August University, Göttingen Germany) on "Performing the New Diasporas: Contemporary African Ritual Music in North America."